THE
MICHELLE WIE
WAY

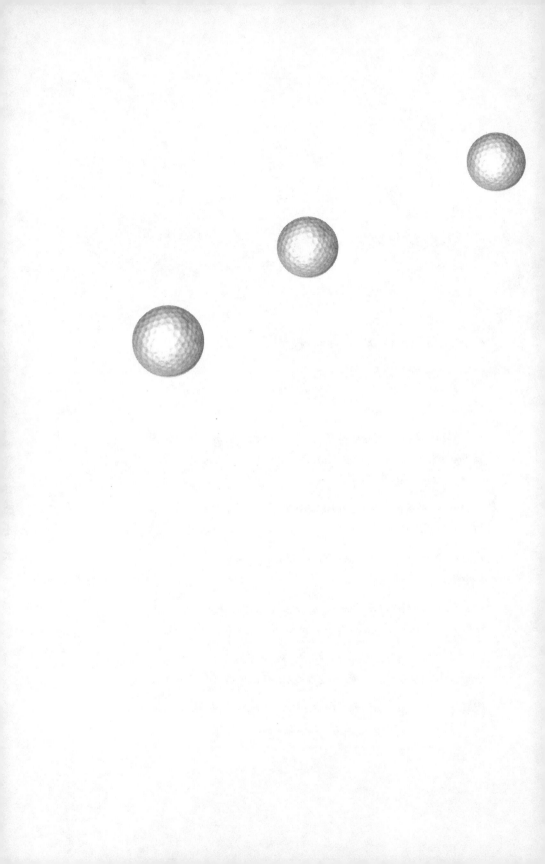

THE
MICHELLE WIE
WAY

Inside Michelle Wie's
Power-Swing Technique

JOHN ANDRISANI

CENTER STREET®

NEW YORK BOSTON NASHVILLE

Grateful acknowledgment is given to Yasuhiro Tanabe
for permission to reprint his photographs.

Center Street

Hachette Book Group USA

237 Park Avenue

New York, NY 10169

Visit our Web site at www.centerstreet.com.

Center Street is a division of Hachette Book Group USA. The Center Street name and logo are trademarks of Hachette Book Group USA.

Printed in the United States of America

First Edition: April 2007

10 9 8 7 6 5 4 3 2 1

Library of Congress Cataloging-in-Publication Data

Andrisani, John.

The Michelle Wie way : inside Michelle Wie's power-swing technique / John Andrisani. — 1st ed.

p. cm.

ISBN-13: 978-1-59995-676-3

ISBN-10: 1-59995-676-4

1. Swing (Golf)   2. Wie, Michelle.   I. Title.

GV979.S9M5 2007

796.352'3—dc222

2006026500

I dedicate this book to Michelle Wie, the teenage golf superstar whose extraordinary power-swing techniques and exceptional all-around shotmaking game are already making their mark on golf history, so much so that I believe wholeheartedly that she is the ultimate new model swinger for male and female golfers to emulate now and well into the future.

ACKNOWLEDGMENTS

The fact that I'm listed as the author of *The Michelle Wie Way* should in no way indicate to you that putting this instructional book together and publishing it was a singular effort. Several individuals deserve credit for the finished product.

I thank my agent Farley Chase of the Waxman Agency for his patience and perseverance in coordinating the contractual details with the book's publisher, Center Street, a division of the Hachette Book Group in New York City.

For help in relaying the clearest, most concise instructional message to readers such as you, I owe gratitude to photographer Yasuhiro Tanabe, whose wonderfully candid "shots" show Michelle Wie's power-swing techniques.

I'm grateful to Chris Park, my talented editor at Center Street. It's befitting that a woman offer me intelligent guidance on writing a book about such a great female golfer as Michelle Wie. I'm also appreciative of the fine work done by Sarah Sper in coordinating this exciting publishing project.

I owe thanks, too, to legendary pros, such as long hitter John Daly and swing aficionado Johnny Miller, and top golf instructors, most notably Jim McLean and Jim Hardy, for the technical knowledge they passed on to me. Their insights better enabled me to analyze Michelle Wie's dynamic, powerful, controlled driver swing, and to pass along to you what I believe are her setup secrets and magical backswing and downswing movements for hitting 300-yard drives and other power shots.

Last, but by no means least, I thank David Leadbetter, Michelle Wie's coach. David and I go way back to the 1980s, when I was *Golf Magazine*'s senior editor and he was one of our publication's teaching editors whom I worked with on instructional articles. And the education I received attending a David Leadbetter Golf Academy instructional school at Champions Gate near Orlando, Florida, served as the strongest foundation for helping me understand the ins and outs of David's teaching method, which continues to have so much to do with the success of Michelle Wie—to me, the greatest swinger of a golf club in the world today.

CONTENTS

THE
MICHELLE WIE
WAY

INTRODUCTION

I was more passionate and excited about writing this instructional book than any of my previous books, including *The Tiger Woods Way*, published in 1997 when Tiger Woods was swinging very differently than he does these days and, as statistics now show, hitting more fairways when driving. Ironically, there is a distinct similarity between Tiger's old power-driving technique and Michelle Wie's present swing, taught to her originally by her father and since 2003 by David Leadbetter, a coach known for possessing a great eye for the fine points of golf technique and for being able to tweak an action and make it more efficient, much in the same way an exceptionally talented mechanic enhances the performance of a Ferrari engine.

I believe Wie's driver swing is technically better than the one Woods employed, so I admit to being a little nervous when

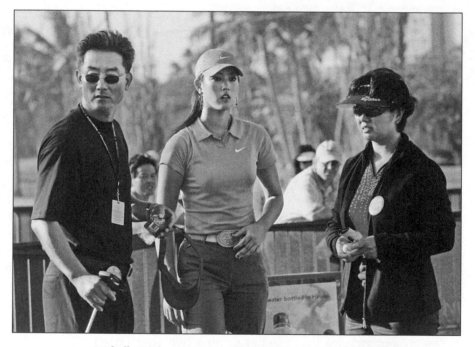

Michelle Wie's winning combination of parental support (top), a strong golf swing (right, top), and a sweet smile (right, bottom) make her a marketing dream-teen for the William Morris Agency and sponsors.

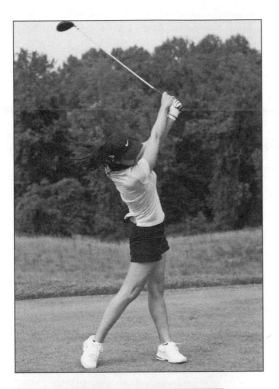

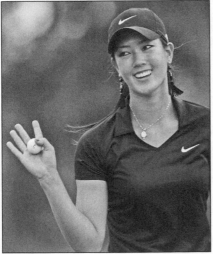

I sat down to write this book. In fact, I felt like what an experienced diamond cutter must feel like when examining a spectacular stone of a rare pink shade found only in South African mines. I make this comparison because when I watched Michelle Wie's swing and analyzed photographs of her extraordinary shotmaking techniques, I experienced a sense of wonderment. At the same time, I felt a heavy weight on my shoulders, knowing it was my job to scrutinize this teenager's swing and reveal to you the reason it stands out and sparkles more than all others in the golf galaxy.

For Johnny Miller, the former Masters and United States Open champion, golf analyst for NBC television, and a no-holds-barred, call-it-like-it-is critic, to comment that "Michelle Wie has one of the best top-five swings of all time" is really saying something. What's more, golf aficionado Greg Hood said, "I never thought I'd see a woman golfer swing better than the great Mickey Wright, and like Ben Hogan hit quality drive after drive." This is a profound statement when you consider that Hood was Hogan's personal assistant, and, more important, that Hogan has long been considered the all-time greatest ball striker and control player, both off the tee and when hitting fairway shots.

Golfer Michelle Wie has been called everything from a child prodigy to golf phenomenon to golfing genius, as if she were born with the talent to hit super-long drives and a wide variety of other creative on-target power shots. In fact, in addition to being blessed with good genes passed down to her from Korean parents, father B.J. and mother Bo, Wie has worked darn hard to evolve into the most exciting player to hit the links since Tiger Woods stepped onto the international golf stage.

Michelle Wie is tall, talented, and so appealing that she is a marketing dream-teen, which is obviously why the William Morris Agency decided to represent this sizzling new star, the first golfer ever on their prestigious client list. Placing Michelle high up on the celebrity pedestal usually reserved for A-list actors, William Morris has already locked in multimillion dollar deals with both Nike and Sony. And, if what I've heard is true, additional megabucks contracts with leading automobile, cosmetic, jewelry, blue jean, and watch companies are already on the table. So it seems that golf's "supergirl"—who, reportedly, even has her own physical trainer, image consultant, and sports psychologist—will indeed become what *Fortune* magazine predicts: "sports' next money machine." Wie is such a unique force that if calculated guesstimates prove right, this young Hawaiian native, who has already played with President William Jefferson Clinton and appeared on both *60 Minutes* and the *Late Show with David Letterman* for interviews, could be cashing in on $40 million a year in endorsements.

At the age of four, Michelle learned the basics of golf from her father, just as Tiger Woods did from his dad, the late Earl Woods. Like Tiger, Michelle spent hours and hours a day for years hitting balls on the driving range to perfect her swing and shotmaking skills. Judging from the quality shots Wie hits consistently during play when competing in women's and men's tournaments around the world, she also obviously learned that one secret to becoming good at golf is ingraining vital setup and swing keys into the muscle memory, rather than thinking about each individual movement and mentally connecting the dots. There's a lesson here, folks. Once on the golf course, the subconscious mind, not the conscious mind, must control the swing action, so that the entire start-to-finish motion flows rhythmically and operates essentially on automatic pilot. In short, although a swing can constantly be tweaked to improve it, once you understand the basic mechanics intellectually, perfect each element through practical practice sessions, and develop a complete flowing motion, you should play by feel.

Though B. J. Wie and renowned coach David Leadbetter have surely helped Michelle Wie evolve into an exceptional golfer, she also obviously had a lot to do with this process. There's no doubt that Wie was born gifted, yet on her own, through trial and error, she learned that all true masters—whether Pablo Picasso, Arthur Rubinstein, Michael Jordan, Muhammad Ali, F. Scott Fitzgerald, or Tiger Woods—go outside the box of basic schooling and add personal nuances to their technique, and that's how they develop a style all their own and rise above their contemporaries. This is where the genius of Michelle Wie lies and why, at just seventeen, she can look back at some incredible accomplishments.

2000: At age ten, Wie shot a score of 64 and also became the youngest player to qualify for the Women's Amateur Public Links Championship.

2001: Won the Hawaii State Women's Stroke Play Championship.

2002: Became the youngest player to qualify for an LPGA tournament and also won the women's division of the Hawaii State Open by 13 strokes.

2003: Won the Women's Amateur Public Links Championship (the youngest winner ever) and finished ninth in her first LPGA major, the Kraft Nabisco Championship.

2004: Won her singles match en route to helping the American team capture the Curtis Cup against their Great Britain & Ireland amateur counterparts, and also finished fourth in the LPGA's Kraft Nabisco Championship.

2005: Finished second to Annika Sorenstam at the LPGA Championship; shot 70 and 71 (one under par) at the PGA Tour John Deere Classic, to miss the cut by only two strokes in an all-male golfer field; reached the quarterfinals of the (traditionally men's) U.S. Amateur Public Links Championship; finished second in the Evian Masters; turned professional at age fifteen, on Wednesday October 5, and on October 13 made her pro debut at the Samsung World Championship, at Bighorn Golf Club in Palm Desert, California.

2006: Playing in her first major championship as a professional—the LPGA Kraft Nabisco Championship—the sixteen-year-old "Tigress" missed getting into a play-off by one shot. However, Wie silenced those critics who claimed she had turned professional too early by finishing third behind winner Karrie Webb, a World Hall of Fame member, and Mexican starlet Lorena Ochoa, who both, incredibly, eagled the par-5 18th hole in the final round.

Wie surprised the golf world by shooting rounds of 70 and 69 to make the cut in the SK Telecom Open, an all-men pro tournament played in Asia.

Michelle also amazed galleries six-deep at New Jersey's Canoe Brook Golf Club, when in June 2006 she shot 68 and 75 to come fairly close to qualifying for the men's United States Open championship.

In the 2006 LPGA championship, Wie's power game was really on. Yet she missed equaling the low 72-hole score by two strokes, owing to some misjudged wedge shots and missed short putts.

Wie tied for third place in the 2006 U.S. Women's Open championship.

Average players who struggle every day to improve at golf are awestruck by Michelle Wie's talents on the course. At tournaments, galleries of golf nuts flock to watch this teenager play. Naturally, since the majority of golfers are obsessed with distance, they come to observe Wie drive the ball in the hope that they will discover a single technical key to picking up extra yards off the tee.

The same level of curiosity, if not more, surrounds Wie's power-swing technique as it did Tiger's initially when he turned professional and was winning major championships by as many as twelve strokes—and with good reason. Golfers can see that Wie generates a tremendous amount of power and looks effortless swinging a golf club.

The main focal point of this book is natural power: secrets to hitting long drives by swinging the club with super efficiency, and picking up extra carry and roll by hitting a high power-draw drive—the Michelle Wie Way.

What do amateur golfers enjoy most about this game, and what drives them to play with such ardent enthusiasm? You'll hear a variety of different answers: the challenge to match par, the excitement of competition, the camaraderie with playing partners, or being outdoors amid the natural beauty that golf courses offer. All of these enjoyable elements are good reasons to play golf. However, the majority of golfers who cite any of the aforementioned reasons for teeing the ball up on a weekend are not admitting the most visceral truth: *It is the universal desire of all golfers to hit the ball a long way.* That's one big reason why Michelle Wie is such an attraction at golf tournaments. No female golfer hits what golfing legend and television commentator Judy Rankin calls "eye-popping tee shots" as often as Wie.

Whether they'll admit it or not, amateur golfers would rather hit long drives than implement any other single improvement in their games. This desire covers the full range of male and female golfers with low, middle range, or high handicaps. Every player in the world gets excited by a long drive and loves to boast about how far they hit the ball on a particular hole when they return to the 19th hole for a beverage after the round. Long drives, more than any other shot played during a round of golf, keeps golfers coming back to the course. Furthermore, past and present golfing greats agree that if you can't drive the ball powerfully and accurately, you can't play good golf.

The golfer's egocentric needs aside, increased power will prove a definite asset to any player at any level. The longer the golfer can drive the ball while keeping it relatively straight, the shorter the iron left to the green, which increases the player's chances of hitting an approach shot within birdie range. Furthermore, in match play competitions, the player who hits powerful drives carries a huge psychological advantage over an opponent onto every tee, as Tiger Woods, John Daly, and Michelle Wie have proven.

The amateur's search for increased power is an ongoing

obsession. To gain an extra ten to twenty yards, he or she takes expensive lessons from big-name pros, reads instructional article after instructional article, watches golf videotapes and DVDs, and swings weighted clubs all winter.

The greatest beneficiary of this quest for power is the golf equipment industry. Because power sells, major golf companies produce power-enhancing items such as drivers with oversize club heads, club shafts constructed of exotic materials like titanium, graphite, and boron, extra-long drivers for a bigger swing arc, and specially designed golf balls with creative aerodynamic dimple patterns that promise to zoom off the club face.

The golfing population's fixation with the power game is, I think, the primary reason why Michelle Wie captures the imagination of galleries everywhere she plays. Wie's appearances in professional tournaments prompt ticket sales and television ratings to rise 50 percent! Golfers just love to watch this teenager hit her signature super-high, super-long, right-to-left soft-draw drive, power-fade tee shot, or hard hit, dead straight tee-ball and listen to the ball flying through the air.

"The sound of Michelle's ball strike is unlike anything I've heard from a female golfer," said Wie's coach David Leadbetter in a *Golf Digest* article.

Wie usually hits a power-draw off the tee, whereas Tiger Woods and most of his fellow PGA Tour players usually hit a power-fade. Wie promotes length through a wide arc of swing, exceptionally good balance, a high degree of hand-arm speed, and a well-timed body-club release in the hitting area. What's more, Wie's action is right-sided, unlike Woods, who is now a left-sided swinger. This is the main reason she typically hits a high powerful draw that lands on the fairway and rolls farther due to increased overspin being imparted on the ball. It's this power-draw shot that will give Wie the best chance of dominating women's golf and even beating male professional golfers at their own game when competing against them in PGA tournaments.

Another plus of Wie's swing is that she hits the ball long without having to create nearly as much club-head speed as long-hitting male professionals. Please don't get me wrong—Wie generates phenomenal speed. On average, Wie's club zooms through the impact zone at around 107 miles per hour. All the same, Wie, like all experienced golf professionals, obviously knows that club speed is not the be-all end-all factor for hitting strong tee shots. To hit the ball powerfully and accurately, the center of the club face must make contact with the center back portion of the ball. Wie is known for contacting the ball with the "sweet spot" of the club face time after time. She also employs a very evenly timed swing, another link to hitting controlled, powerful drives.

Through my analysis, golfers will get the insight they've been looking for from Wie's methods of hitting powerful tee shots and, in addition, explanations of how she plays a variety of other on-target power shots during a round of golf.

What sets this instructional book apart from others is it goes beyond simply discussing all-important fundamentals, and includes nuances of Wie's technique that all golfers should take the time to learn. For example, emulating Wie's trigger-finger grip will help you discover a new source of power and control. Copying the way Wie rotates her shoulders to the maximum and minimizes her hip turn motion will enable you to increase what's called the backswing's X-Factor differential, and thus program added power into your action—provided that, like Wie, you also create a wide arc of swing by extending your arms and the club back as far as is comfortably possible in the takeaway. Furthermore, if like Wie you learn to trigger the downswing with your right side, and also drive the lower body toward the target while the upper body tilts back away from it in the hitting area, you will have cracked the code to solving the mystery of contacting the ball powerfully on the upswing with the center of the driver's club face.

Through in-depth analysis of Wie's driver-swing technique and by examining the color sequence photographs in the insert, you will discover the uniqueness of Wie's address, backswing, and downswing. All elements of Wie's technique are impressive, yet what I'd like you to pay closest attention to is the second half of this superstar's swing.

Michelle's downswing operates much like a player piano. Once the instrument is turned on, it plays a melodic tune automatically. Similarly, once Wie's right side "fires" at the start of the downswing, Wie swings melodically through all the paramount positions without consciously tinkling the keys. This will be good news to millions of frustrated golfers who make the mistake of depending too much on the left side of their body, rather than their natural right side to trigger the downswing, and try consciously to direct the club into the ball on the downswing, rather than letting the swing simply happen according to the laws of physics, namely centrifugal force.

Another feature of Michelle Wie's swing that you've likely witnessed is her incredible rhythm. It's an understatement to call it smooth; *powerfully poetic* better describes Wie's effortless-looking swing motion.

Chances are, you know the truth deep down in your heart: you fail to hit good tee shots consistently because you swing so fast that you lose your balance. Though Michelle Wie obviously knows the importance of generating sufficient club-head speed to compress the ball, she demonstrates that the real secret to hitting long drives is "club-head speed correctly applied," in the words of teaching legend John Jacobs from England. What does this mean? The tempo of your swing can be fast, as long as you remain balanced enough in the hitting area to return the club face squarely to the ball. Lots of weekend golfers are strong and generate high club-head speed, yet they swing so fast that they fail to co-ordinate the movement of the body with the movement of the club in a synchronized manner. Consequently, they hit the ball long but off line. But Wie's club-head speed is controlled; this is so because coach David Leadbetter stresses the importance of swinging the driver with *manageable acceleration.*

Ideally, reading the instructional commentary and looking at the photographs of Wie's swing in this book will encourage you to discipline yourself to concentrate on club-head smoothness rather than sheer club-head speed, and to learn the art of developing a flowing rhythmic action. Once you do, during a round of golf, you'll be able to hit a variety of power shots that land on the fairway or close to the flagstick.

I trust you are as excited about reading this book as I was researching and writing it, so let's go to the practice tee and participate together in a lesson program, starting with how to set up to hit powerful drives. We'll then move on to the secrets for programming power into your backswing, learn how to unleash power on the downswing and, finally, focus on how to increase your scoring potential by becoming educated on the art of hitting a variety of powerful shots from on and off the fairway.

John Andrisani
Gulfport, Florida

SETTING UP TO RIP IT!

Michelle Wie's winning combination of proven fundamentals and personal setup nuances works wonders when it comes to consistently producing super-powerful, super-accurate tee shots

M ichelle Wie may well be established as the prototype for the professional woman golfer of the future. Tall and blessed with athletic talent, Michelle dominates courses by hitting drives over the 300-yard mark quite regularly and averaging at least 280 yards. While this distance is unheard-of for a female player, Wie is likely to get longer—substantially longer—in the next several years, since her frame will naturally fill out. It's no stretch at all to suggest that Wie will soon average at least 300 yards off the tee, making her longer than all but the longest hitters on the men's PGA Tour.

One key to Wie's long-hitting prowess is unquestionably the extremely large, wide arc that she is able to create and maintain, especially when swinging the driver. Obviously,

Wie's height of 6′ 1″ and long arms, along with the flexibility that comes with still being a teenager, help her accomplish this technical link to producing powerful tee shots. Having said that, her extraordinary length can mostly be attributed to a near-perfect overall technique. More than one of the world's golf-swing gurus, most notably Johnny Miller, have ranked Michelle's golf swing among the top five in the world. On the surface, ranking a seventeen-year-old girl's golf swing right up there with the likes of Tiger Woods, Ben Hogan, and Sam Snead borders on the absurd. However, if you are a student of the game and have watched Michelle Wie in action on the golf course, you know these experts are absolutely correct in their assessments.

Wie's height advantage over almost all her other female competitors is following a trend on the men's PGA Tour. In reference to the men professionals, it was long thought that golfers of medium height, or even slightly shorter than medium height, were likely to make the best golfers. The theory was that a medium-size player would be better able to keep himself and the club moving under control than the taller player, who might struggle more to maintain good balance and control of the swing. Numerous examples have supported this view, such as champions Ben Hogan, Gary Player, Lee Trevino, and Tom Watson.

However, golf at the very highest level has changed dramatically, even since the mid-1990s. The top male professionals now hit the ball with such power that they are making some of the finest tests of golf in the world virtually obsolete. Improved equipment, of course, has played a huge role in this metamorphosis. But the size and athletic ability of today's top male golfers is inarguably the prime reason that golf has become such a power game. It is certainly no coincidence that the top five golfers in the world at the time of writing—Tiger Woods, Phil Mickelson, Vijay Singh, Retief Goosen, and Ernie Els—are all well over six feet tall (Els, at 6′ 4″, is the tallest). All of these golfers, especially Woods and Singh, are also noted for their intense devotion to physical training and fitness.

Although there is no doubt that women professional golfers are also getting bigger and stronger, it is probably fair to say that their raw athletic skills have not surged as rapidly as the men's. Michelle Wie's athletic ability and virtually flawless mechanical technique are likely to set the bar for what the female golf swing can accomplish, in terms of combined distance and accuracy, for some time to come.

An Athletic Setup

No matter how gifted an individual may be in terms of size, strength, suppleness, and coordination, he or she is not likely to go far in the game of golf without repeatedly setting up to the ball correctly.

"A good setup is the most important fundamental in every athletic swing," said David Leadbetter in his instruction book *The Golf Swing.*

Golfing legend Jack Nicklaus was equally profound, making this statement in his best-selling book *Golf My Way*: "If you set up correctly, there's a good chance you'll hit a reasonable shot, even if you make a mediocre swing. If you set up incorrectly, you'll hit a lousy shot even if you make the greatest swing in the world."

Let's now take a close look at how Michelle Wie sets up to the ball with the driver, examining the most vital elements of grip, body and club alignment, ball position, as well as posture. With the exception of a few idiosyncratic elements, Michelle's setup is a classic model for any player who is seeking to hit long, powerful tee shots.

Grip Tips

While a good grip does not guarantee that a player will employ a good golf swing, the correlation between an imperfect grip and a less-than-ideal swing is very high. Michelle Wie holds the club in a way that allows her arms to swing the club along the correct path and plane without having to make any compensatory adjustments with her left hand or right hand during the backswing or downswing. In contrast to the average middle- to high-handicap golfer, whose hands are typically extremely active (a common fault causing errant shots), Wie's hands are passive until she reaches the hitting area.

In most great golf swings, the role of the hands is minimized. In Michelle's case, the hands act solely as the linkage between the player and the club. Her good grip allows her to make a swing that maximizes the use of her large body muscles, rather than the smaller muscles, and thereby enables her to swing the club consistently on the correct path and plane—from start to finish—and hit a high percentage of powerfully accurate drives.

The critical feature of Wie's grip is that both hands are essentially in what is commonly referred to by golf instructors as a "neutral" position. In short, this means that the hands are placed on the handle in a position that enables them to work with, rather than against, each other and return the club face square to the ball at the point of impact. Let's look at this position in detail.

Michelle begins her grip by placing the club somewhat diagonally across the palm of her left hand. The butt of the grip is just beyond the base of the palm, and the grip runs up diagonally across the palm and covers the first joint of her index finger. As she closes this hand, the club's handle is snugly secured between the butt of the palm and the last three fingers of the left hand. Her left index finger is slightly separated from her other three fingers; this bit of space will allow for the linking of the right hand with the left in the completed grip. Meanwhile, Michelle's left thumb, when closed over the top of the grip, rests just to the right of the top-center of the club's handle. When her left-hand grip is thus completed, she can see the top knuckle on both her index and middle fingers, but no more than that. The V-shape made by the inside lines of her left thumb and index finger points upward, virtually midway between her chin and right shoulder.

Next, Michelle inserts the little finger of her right hand into the gap between her left index and middle fingers. The right little finger works underneath the left index finger, rather than resting atop the finger. Thus, Michelle is using an interlock rather than the more traditional overlapping, or Vardon, style of grip. The choice of an interlocking or overlapping grip is more a matter of personal preference than a fundamental—it is the positioning of both the hands in relation to the club's grip, and by extension their relationship to the position of the club face, that is the most crucial element of a good grip. That said, although the interlock grip is still used by a minority of golfers when compared to the overlap, there seems to be an increasing trend toward the use of the interlock, as it serves to knit the hands together more securely. Tiger Woods, the world's number-one golfer and winner of twelve major championships, uses an interlocking grip, as did Jack Nicklaus en route to winning a record eighteen majors during his long professional career. Expect the same kind of success from Michelle Wie.

After interlocking the little finger of her right hand, Michelle places her ring and middle fingers underneath the grip, then folds the palm of her right hand securely over her left thumb. The club's handle is thus locked between the upward pressure of the middle two fingers of her right hand, and the pressure from the palm above. Michelle's right thumb rests on the top left of the grip, with the inside of that thumb and the inside of her right index finger also applying a slight pinching pressure to the grip. In the completed right-hand position, the V formed between the right thumb and right forefinger also points approximately to an area between her chin and right shoulder.

Michelle's grip puts her hands in a classic, neutral position on the club. This is the position in which it is most natural for the hands to return at impact.

If Michelle's hands were turned farther to the right on the handle (in what is known as a "strong" position) she would have to fight the tendency to return the club face into a closed position at impact. If you look at the grips of amateur golfers, you will see that many recreational players hold the club with the hands turned into this strong position. Precisely why this is the case, I cannot say for sure— perhaps this position gives the player the sense that he or she can control the club better and hit the ball longer. However, the opposite is true. Strong-grip players often have to deal with spells of hitting uncontrollable weak duck-hook shots that dart left of target practically the split-second the club face contacts the ball.

If, on the other hand, Michelle's hands were turned farther to the left (in what's known as a "weak" position), she would need to employ an extra, artificial flipping movement with the hands through impact in order to keep the club face from remaining open at impact and hitting a slice, a shot that flies well right of target and is the most common among high-handicap male and female amateur players. Because Michelle's hands are in a natural, neutral position, almost as they would be when at rest at her sides, she does not need to rely on any hand manipulation during the swing. Instead, Michelle's hands merely go along for the ride until she enters the impact zone, when they snap the club face into the ball.

Tailoring the Tip

It is easy for any amateur or pro golfer to suddenly develop a bad grip habit. So, when gripping the golf club, be conscious of positioning the palm of the right hand parallel to the palm of your left hand. It's also prudent to have your grip checked periodically by your local golf professional or to take your address in front of a mirror to be sure the Vs of your grip are correct. Today, at many public and private clubs, you'll find at least one mirror on the practice range.

There are two other points about Michelle's grip that might be considered idiosyncratic. One is that her left thumb, which you cannot see in the completed grip, is stretched fully down the club's handle. This "long thumb" position (as opposed to a "short thumb," which is somewhat cinched up on the grip) provides extra support for the weight of the club as it reaches the top of the backswing.

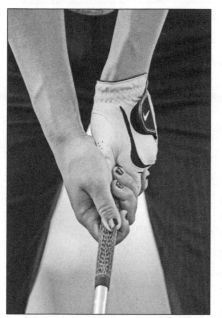

Michelle Wie uses the same interlocking grip as Tiger Woods, yet her idiosyncratic left hand "long thumb" and right hand "trigger finger" help her hit powerfully accurate shots.

In my opinion, it also gives Michelle a little more leverage from underneath the club, in getting it started back down toward the ball. If you have never thought about this aspect of the grip, and a great many golfers have not, check to see if you can extend your left thumb a bit farther down the handle. You will probably like that feeling of a little better support of the club.

The other slight idiosyncrasy of Michelle's grip is how she drapes her right index finger under the club's handle and keeps it separated from her middle finger. This "trigger finger" position is a trait that she shares with John Daly, and with Lee Trevino and Johnny Miller in their prime years. It's doubtful that Michelle was specifically taught to adopt this unorthodox position; she likely adapted it herself through experimentation in practice or by noticing it when studying the grips of those great players mentioned.

The trigger finger, however arrived at, seems to have two things going for it. First, it can enhance the golfer's feel for the club head. This heightened sense of feel no doubt helped Trevino to become the greatest player of his era at shaping shots; and, for Miller, it may have contributed to the uncanny distance control he exhibited with his irons when he went on his big winning streaks. Second, the trigger position can provide the golfer with an added degree of freedom and power when releasing the driver in the hitting area. This sure is true in the case of power hitter John Daly, who told me the idiosyncratic trigger position "gives the club shaft a little bit of extra snap coming through impact."

Your Lesson

The trigger-finger approach, being something big hitters such as Wie and Daly employ, could be an element that you or any other amateur in search of more distance off the tee might want to consider.

Alignment Tips

Once she has established her grip, then angled her club toward the target, and stared at an ideal area of fairway to

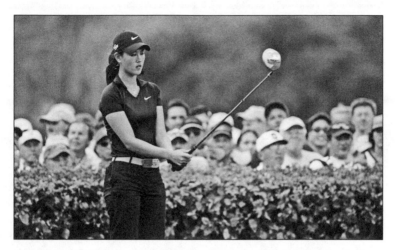

Standing behind the ball and pointing the club at the target is part of Michelle's pre-swing routine that helps her step into the shot correctly, with her body and club face aligned properly.

land the ball, Michelle Wie steps into the "golfer's box" with correct alignment her priority.

Depending on the type of drive Michelle plans to hit, her alignment changes accordingly.

For example, if Michelle's objective is to hit a dead-straight tee shot, imaginary lines running across her feet, knees, hips, and shoulders are parallel to yet another imaginary line running from the ball to the target. The club face is positioned perpendicular to the target, usually a small area of grass in the center of the fairway. The best way to promote a "square" setup is to imagine a railroad track with one rail representing the body line, the other the ball-target line.

While on the subject of the straight shot, I will mention a nuance in Wie's setup that I found very interesting.

Michelle sets the club down about one inch back from the ball itself. The great Ben Hogan did something very similar to this, only he set the club down two inches behind the ball. Either way, this unorthodox setup element will help you employ a low, extended takeaway action that, in turn, will serve as a catalyst in triggering a wide, powerful swing arc.

When hitting her bread-and-butter power-draw drive, Michelle aims just slightly right of target, with her setup marked by a "closed stance"—a term used to describe a position in which the right foot is a couple of inches farther away from the target line than the left foot. This type of stance will provide you with a feeling of added freedom in

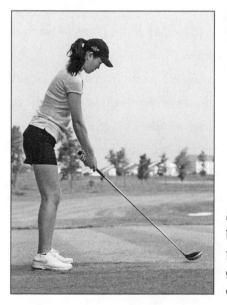

Most of the time Michelle sets her feet slightly "closed," in preparation for hitting her go-to shot: the power-draw drive.

swinging the club along an inside path and will promote a shot that curves a little to the left in the air or "draws" toward a target in the fairway.

At times, when she's required to hit a power-fade (a shot that turns quietly to the right in the air and one that will be covered in chapter 4), Michelle sets her feet and body left of target, along the line on which the ball will start flying, and the club at the point where she expects the ball to come to rest, usually down the right portion of fairway on a dogleg right hole (hole curves quite dramatically to the right).

Proper Ball Position

One other element of the setup that is crucial to attaining power and accuracy off the tee is the position of the ball in relation to the stance. A player can set up with perfect alignment, but still hit the ball consistently off line if the ball is not positioned correctly in relation to the body. If the ball is too far forward, the club face will have started to close at impact, so that the right-handed player will pull or hook the shot. When the ball is too far back, the player will either push or slice the shot, because the club face will tend not to return to a square position. With the driver, Michelle positions the ball opposite a line drawn to the inside of her left armpit. This positioning allows her to return the club face to square at impact without any artificial manipulations, and it also allows her to contact the ball with the club face just as it begins to ascend from the bottom of its arc, something we'll discuss at further length later.

Tips on Posture

Many tall golfers struggle to maintain a comfortable and balanced posture over the ball. However, Michelle Wie, no doubt with great tutelage from her father, B.J., and present coach David Leadbetter, has developed a posture that is exemplary. If you compare Michelle's setup photos with those of Tiger Woods in my book *The Tiger Woods Way*, which were taken at about the time he turned pro in 1996, you will find an awful lot of similarities between the two.

As befitting a tall player using a driver, Michelle, like Tiger, takes a wide stance—the distance between her heels is about four inches wider than the outside edge of her shoulders. This is a little wider than most teachers might advocate, but Michelle's extended base makes it much easier for her to develop a super-wide swing arc for maximum power. I like seeing this feature of Michelle's setup, especially since former U.S. Open champion Ken Venturi, for whom I have a tremendous amount of respect, made it clear to me on several occasions that a wide base is the only way to establish a strong foundation for swinging the club powerfully and maintaining balance in the impact zone.

While Michelle's right foot points outward about 20 degrees from the perpendicular position, as is typical among top players, her left foot is only very slightly toed-out, per-haps only 5 degrees from a right angle to the target line. This left-foot positioning in particular differs from both the recommendation of most teachers and the practice of most legendary golfers, including Woods, Nicklaus, Hogan, and Snead. For all these players, the left foot is toed out by about a 30-degree angle. The theory behind this placement of the left foot is that the toed-out position makes it easier for the player to turn his or her hips fully and freely counterclock-wise through and past impact.

The natural question on every golfer's mind: Is Wie, tech-nically speaking, making an error in keeping her left foot nearly perpendicular to the target line? Given the results she is getting, she appears to be instinctively doing the right thing, at least at this early stage of her career. Michelle is so flexible that keeping the left foot straight does not hamper her ability to turn her lower torso through the shot very much at all, as we will see when we discuss the downswing. Meanwhile, by keeping her left foot nearly squared up (much like Sergio Garcia, who generates tremendous power for his size) Michelle is much less likely to let her left leg bow outward or sag through the impact zone. Instead, she is set up to unleash the power of her right side against a firm left leg, something that John Daly also does very well when booming drives down the fairway. If the positioning of your left or front foot is something that you have not considered, it is certainly something worth experimenting with on the practice tee. If you are fairly flexible, you may find that a straight left foot—and the firm left side "wall" it helps you build and turn around in the hitting area—will add some power to your shots. If you are not flexible, perhaps toeing your left foot out a little more than you usually do will encourage a freer turn of your lower torso through impact.

Two other things stand out regarding Michelle's posture:

1. Michelle's entire head and most of her body are behind the ball at address. Since she is already essentially behind the ball (with about 55 to 60 percent of her weight on her right foot), she does not need to slide her body weight farther to the right as she swings her arms, hands, and the club back. Rather, she can concentrate on turning away from the ball. This head and body position thus encourages good balance, and helps keep the club on-plane during the backswing.

2. The shaft of Michelle's driver is angled back somewhat from the bottom of the shaft up to the grip. This means that Michelle's hands are a few inches behind the ball at address. Most amateurs have the club shaft leaning forward and their hands ahead of the ball at address. As I recollect, before Michelle began learning from David Leadbetter, her hands were ahead of the club face, albeit only slightly. The problem with this hands-ahead position, especially if exaggerated, is that it encourages you

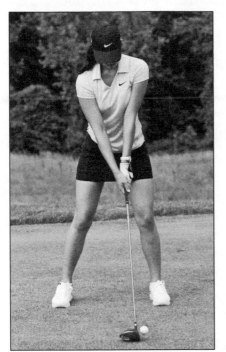

From this front view angle, you can clearly see Michelle's unorthodox hands-behind-ball position.

to pull the club up quickly on an overly steep angle and ultimately hit fat irons and slices off the tee.

It is somewhat unusual, however, for a player's hands to be behind the ball at address. In this regard, though, Wie is in very good company: both Ben Hogan and Tiger Woods (perhaps more so at the beginning of his pro career when he was hitting the ball more accurately than he is at present) favored the hands-back setup. By starting with the hands a bit behind the ball, Michelle is encouraged to push the club back longer along the target line, creating the beginning of what will be a very wide swing arc. At the same time, it is virtually impossible to jerk the club sharply upward or whip the club head way inside the target line when you start with the hands slightly behind the ball. For these reasons, this is another aspect of Wie's setup you should try to emulate.

Michelle's posture at address demonstrates an exceptional degree of balance and readiness. Her weight is distributed equally between the balls and the heels of her feet, so she is neither leaning in toward nor back from the ball.

Michelle's knees are flexed, but not deeply bent, so that her kneecaps are directly above the balls of her feet and her rear end is just slightly behind a line drawn to the backs of her heels. This is what David Leadbetter refers to as the "ready" position: It is the balanced posture of athletes in many other sports, such as a baseball infielder as a pitch is being thrown to a batter, or a basketball player who is ready to guard the ball handler for the opposing team. In golf, instead of being ready to react to the movements of opposing players, the player is ready to put her own movements into motion, starting from an extremely well-balanced position.

Wie also bends forward from her hips, rather than from her waist. By bending from her hips, Michelle's entire spine is bent forward uniformly, as opposed to having her upper back and shoulders slumped forward more than the lower half of her spine. This uniform bending of her back makes it much easier for her to make a pure turn of the body about her spine, something that every golfer should emulate.

As Michelle bends forward, she is still in a fairly erect posture. She bends her spine forward by about a 30-degree angle, which is not a tremendous amount of spine bend for a tall player. This will prove beneficial as she executes her backswing turn; it sets her up to swing on a plane or angle that is not too steep, something that we will discuss in detail in the next chapter.

Michelle also positions her hands well away from her body, perhaps a little more than the hand-width distance that most teachers recommend. Because she is reaching with her arms just a trifle, there is a very wide angle between the arms and the club shaft. The average golfer, who is usually much too tense at address, would be well advised to allow his or her arms to hang down in a relaxed fashion like Michelle's and to also copy her way of creating a larger gap between the hands and body. Both of these setup tips will allow you to make a free, accelerating swing.

Michelle Wie's setup contains the perfect mix of proven fundamentals and personal nuances to promote a power swing. Michelle's setup is one that any handicap amateur would do well to copy to the letter. To echo the thoughts of Jack Nicklaus regarding grip, alignment, and posture, if you could learn to set up to all full shots as well as Michelle Wie does, it would be hard not to make a repetitive and powerful golf swing. Consequently, what I advise you to do is spend time rehearsing the elements of Wie's setup. Next, have a friend videotape your address from both the face-on and down-target angles. Developing a balanced and athletic setup like Michelle's will make the development of an athletic, powerful swing motion much more attainable. In the next section, which analyzes Michelle Wie's backswing, you can begin to do just that.

MICHELLE WIE'S MASTERFUL SETUP POSITIONS

Michelle uses an interlock grip, the same unified way of holding the club upon which Jack Nicklaus and Tiger Woods have depended throughout their careers. In this grip, the little finger of the right hand is linked underneath the index finger of the left hand in the completed hold on the club. An increasing number of tour professionals are now following Michelle's example and using this type of grip, claiming that it enhances their control of the club throughout the swing.

Michelle's flat and long left thumb position programs control into the swing. Her right forefinger "trigger" is a definite power source; it helps her snap the club into the ball through impact at a high speed of around 107 miles per hour.

Michelle positions her hands slightly behind the ball when setting up to drive, a trait she shares with the late Ben Hogan, the legendary powerful and consistent driver and fairway shotmaker. Setting up with the hands in this position virtually guarantees that Michelle will drag the club head straight back from the ball (while keeping it low to the ground), commencing a swing with the widest possible arc.

Michelle's stance with the driver is wide; the distance between the insides of her heels is about four inches wider than the width of her shoulders. The wider stance provides a stable base to support her powerful upper body turn and strong movement through the ball on the downswing.

Michelle exaggerates the upper tilt of her left hip at address. This setup nuance allows her to be poised to hit the ball powerfully on the upswing.

HOW TO PROGRAM POWER INTO THE BACKSWING

Michelle Wie's unique body turn and the wide arc of swing she creates
are vital links to hard-hit, on-target shots

Michelle Wie employs what may go down as the finest and most powerful golf swings up to this point in golf history. However, as you are likely an average club golfer who has probably been tempted to give up the game at least once during your life, it's important to realize that the swing you see in this book is not the swing that Michelle Wie was born with. Granted, Wie is blessed physically, particularly when it comes to innate strength, flexibility, and hand-eye coordination. Still, much of the nearly perfect form Michelle displays on the golf course has been developed, adjusted, and improved, mostly through hard work over the past several years with Leadbetter.

At this point, I'm sure some of you are saying, "It's all well and good to have all this raw talent, and have David Leadbetter, probably the most sought-after teacher in the world, to constantly coach you. I don't have access to a swing coach like that, so how can I make swing corrections the way I need to?" My answer: You have in this book a "blueprint" comprised of words and pictures designed to help you develop a technically sound power-golf swing by using Michelle Wie as your ultimate model-professional.

Generating Power from "Inside-Out"

Before discussing the specific movements of Wie's backswing, it is important for you to understand this big-picture tenet of the modern golf swing: *Power that is transferred into speed in the club head at impact is developed primarily by the turning of the torso as fully as possible around a central point in the backswing, and then releasing this stored-up energy by re-turning the body in the opposite direction during the downswing.*

In his book *The Golf Swing*, David Leadbetter uses the analogy of a pair of figure skaters performing a spinning display to describe a golfer developing speed in the club head. The lead skater (usually the male in a male-female pair) acts as the pivot or the central point around which the second skater, whose hand he is holding, spins around with dizzying speed. In this way the lead skater is akin to the body during the golf swing, and the second skater is like the club head. The lead skater, who is in a compact, near-sitting position on the ice, starts to rotate slowly around a fixed point. As he does so, the second skater, like the club head, begins to pick up speed. As the central figure begins to turn faster in circles around a fixed point, the second skater revolves around him in a manner that is many times faster. As the performance reaches its climax, the central skater is still moving relatively slowly around a fixed point, but the second skater whips around him with blinding speed. This image shows the power and speed that is generated through centrifugal force: a force generated from an interior, fixed point, transferred to an object that is attached to, and swinging around, this interior point.

Gerald Walford, ranked among the top sixty instructors by the World Golf Teachers Federation, agrees with Leadbetter. He takes the relationship between such scientific principles and the golf swing to a new dimension, and re-iterated to me what he essentially says in his book *Performance Golf*:

> The golf swing is an arc of a circle and is based on a pendulum. The arc of the pendulum swings from the center of the circle. The center of the swing is the top of the left shoulder, while the left arm and the golf club form the

radius. The club's head, while in motion, prescribes the arc of the swing.

Gravity pulls the club down faster from the 9 o'clock position than from the 7 o'clock position. This simple law of the pendulum, discovered by Leonardo da Vinci, means that the longer the backswing and follow-through the faster the club will move and the faster the ball will fly.

In the golf swing, enormous speed in the club head is generated by the comparatively slow turning of the upper torso around a fixed axis—namely, the player's spine. The golfer who turns his or her torso significantly faster than average will be capable of developing tremendous club-head speed. Various top teachers refer to Tiger Woods' tremendous rotational speed—the quickness with which he rotates his body, specifically on the downswing. It is this quickness, rather than brute strength, which translates into his fantastic club-head speed and power at impact.

In addition to the turning of the torso to develop club-head speed, the longer the distance between the center of the player's torso and the club head (which travels on what we call the "arc" of the swing), the greater the amount centrifugal force produced, and the faster, relatively, the club head will move.

Now that I've given you a broad sense of what's involved in generating power, let's look closely at the more intricate details involved in the great game of inches called golf.

Pre-Swing Secrets

For Michelle Wie or any other good player, there is a brief period of time between the point at which the player has completed the setup and is ready to swing, and the start of the swing itself. This is when the player takes his or her final look at the target, makes one or more waggles of the club (i.e., lifts the club up, back, and around behind the ball, usually using wrist motion to do so), looks down at the ball and back at the target one more time, and finally swings.

Golfers go through all sorts of preparations before they finally swing—including lifting and repositioning their feet, gripping and regripping the club, or maybe just standing motionless over the ball for a few seconds until the right feel for triggering the swing clicks in. My point: What you do just before starting the backswing is a reflection of your own personality. Therefore, no good teacher will tell you what you're doing is wrong. Nevertheless, there is a caveat.

While most experts agree that physically going through a simple, standardized routine prior to starting the backswing is far better than stepping into the address and swinging back straight away, Dr. Bob Rotella, a noted sports psychologist, coach to PGA and LPGA Tour pros, and author of *Golf Is Not a Game of Perfect*, points out that any routine that impedes the golfer's focus on the only thing that he or she should have in mind—the target—is bound to be counterproductive.

No doubt Rotella would approve of Michelle Wie's no-nonsense approach to her full shots. Once Michelle sets the club down, feels her body is aligned properly, and finishes her series of ball-to-target glances, she starts the backswing. She does not even waggle the club as most golfers do at address, let alone make any other extraneous movements or freeze over the ball.

This is something all golfers can learn from. Once you have set up to play a shot, both meticulously and correctly, there is no point in standing over the ball while mentally agonizing. All this can do is give you time to think about things other than your target (i.e., trees, water, or technical thoughts regarding some part of the swing). PGA Tour professional Sergio Garcia learned the hard way that "milking" the grip some twenty times before swinging was impairing his concentration and ability to hit good golf shots. Sergio's pre-swing routine is much shorter now and he's starting to see better results.

Your Lesson

Develop a pre-swing routine that is, even if not precisely like Michelle's, one that is prompt and decisive. Granted, you may not have your mechanics exactly where you want them, and they are probably not second nature to you either. Still, from my experience as a former golf teacher, you will give yourself the best chance to swing freely, without inhibition, and hit a solid on-target shot if you avoid dilly-dallying over the ball at address.

Takeaway: Low and Wide

Michelle's address position with the driver, as touched on earlier, is unique because of the way she sets her hands a few inches behind the ball. This setup may be unorthodox, but it promotes a wide takeaway action that creates power more easily.

Once Michelle triggers the backswing by turning her body-center in a clockwise direction, her hands (in response to the movement of the torso rather than by an independent movement of their own), slowly start back from the ball. These movements start occurring a split second before the club head starts to move back. This very slight lag, with the torso and the hands moving before the club head, ensures that the club head will begin its journey by moving slowly and very low to the ground. At the point where Michelle's torso has turned to about 1 o'clock on the clock face and her hands are about even with her right thigh, the club head will have caught up with her body turn and her hands. The club head will then be carried, if you will, all the way up to the top by her hands and arms. Notice that I said that the club is "carried" back by the hands. At this point in the backswing, the hands remain essentially passive. They are merely holding on to the club and carrying it backward and upward in response to Michelle's turning torso.

As Michelle's torso continues to turn and her hands are at hip height, her left arm is fully extended and the club head is beginning to describe a wide arc around her midsection. At this stage of the swing, the club shaft is pointing directly toward the target and the shaft lies above a line that points straight down to the tips of Michelle's toes. Both of these points indicate that the club is being swung around by her body, with little if any hand manipulation. Meanwhile, the toe of Michelle's driver is pointing straight up. Most golfers, teachers included, think of the club's toe-up position at this point in the swing as being perfectly square. In reality, this means that the club face is in a slightly open position. If the club was 100 percent square to the path of the swing, the toe would point more to the right, to about 1 o'clock on an imaginary clock face. What Michelle's club-face position shows is that just prior to reaching this point her forearms have begun to rotate just slightly in a counterclockwise direction. The arms must rotate and the right wrist, which we'll talk about in detail a little later, must cock in order to carry the club up to the top-of-backswing position. The fact that a bit of forearm rotation has occurred by the time Michelle has reached this point in the backswing is certainly not a problem as long as it is not overdone to the point where the club face starts to point more upward. If that were the case, this would indicate a substantial rolling of the forearms, and with them the club head, into an overly open position, which would lead to a very flat plane for the club swing. But as it stands here, Michelle turns and places the club in *the* textbook position at this point of the swinging action.

It should be mentioned here that the position I have just described was apparently not natural or automatic for Wie. It's my understanding that before Michelle first visited David Leadbetter as a thirteen-year-old, she had several back-swing flaws. These included a hands-and-wrists-oriented takeaway in which she cocked the club up and away from the ball at a steep angle. This hands-oriented takeaway was due in part to the fact that at address, her hands were po-sitioned ahead of the ball rather than behind it as they are now. Be that as it may, this hands-oriented takeaway pre-cluded her from getting her torso to turn immediately into the swing as the main power generator and, in turn, caused her to develop a relatively narrow swing arc. Both of these faults resulted in loss of club-head speed and thus power at impact. No doubt as a result of these two flaws, Michelle also did what many women players do—overswing, so that the shaft of the club drops well below parallel to the ground at the top of the backswing. I mention these adjustments to illustrate that there is no such thing as a person who is born with a perfect golf swing. Michelle Wie had to first understand what she was doing in the early portion of her backswing, understand what changes she needed to make, and work on the appropriate movement until it felt natural and easy to repeat over and over again. Michelle obviously has learned a lot, owing to lessons with Leadbetter. Right now, her takeaway is excellent.

It is also a good idea to examine your own takeaway po-

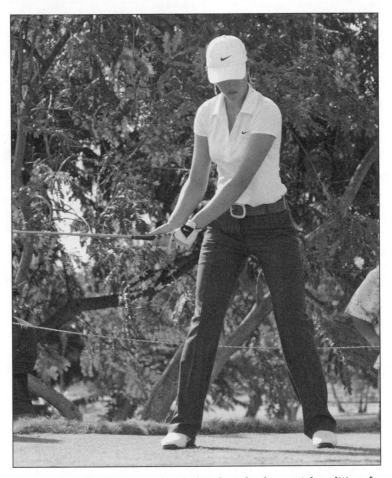

One word—EXTENSION—can be used to describe the special qualities of Michelle Wie's takeaway action. The fact that there's no ball in the picture tells you that Michelle is more interested in rehearsing this vital action than hitting shots.

You too want to create a wide arc of swing and power by extending the club and arms back away from the target. So when practicing these vital features of golf technique, try and feel how the big muscles of your torso, and not those in your hands, control the action.

sition in front of a full-length mirror, and determine the differences between your body, arm, and club positions when compared to Wie's. Since each individual's swing to this point has differing flaws, I cannot advise you on what adjustments you need to make. However, you certainly can look at your original setup position, to see whether it is conducive to excessive hand and wrist movement in the takeaway; you can start learning to feel that you start the takeaway with a turning of the torso; and you can train yourself to keep your left arm well extended to this point in the backswing, to widen your swing arc. Most of all, follow Michelle Wie's example and get your backswing off to a sound start, one that activates the big muscles of your torso and minimizes the role of your hands in the golf swing.

Going Up: Wrists Hinge, Right Knee Stays Firm

Michelle continues to wind her torso fluidly on the backswing; the chief goal being to coil her body-center as far as her degree of flexibility will comfortably allow. At this point in the swing, Michelle's left arm is parallel to the ground while the club shaft is pointing straight up to the sky. In addition, Michelle's torso and shoulders have turned approximately 75 degrees from the position in which she started. For many golfers, even some exceptionally good ones, this degree of shoulder turn is more than they can muster even at the very top of their backswings. Yet, Wie's club shaft will travel yet another 90 degrees up and around to her top-of-backswing position. This degree of shoulder turn at this point in the backswing clearly indicates that Michelle's upper torso is the main generator of her backswing motion.

The club shaft is now virtually at right angles to Michelle's straight left arm. This has occurred because Michelle's wrists hinge or cock upward substantially. This wrist-hinging in the backswing occurs naturally rather than as a consciously thought-out action. Specifically, it happens in response to the turning body, and encourages Michelle to direct the club up from the plane it moved on previously, especially once the right elbow begins folding. We'll talk more about this lifting motion of the arms and the swing plane during the discussion of the top-of-backswing position.

What I need to emphasize is the naturalness of Michelle's "set-action" of the wrists. This is not a conscious movement. You can feel this for yourself by taking a club and setting it in the halfway-back position, so that the club shaft is pointing away from the target. In order to complete the backswing from here, you *must* begin to flex your right elbow upward—if you didn't, your backswing would come to a halt with the club still pointed more or less behind you, with your left arm pointing straight back and with virtually no wrist hinge. So, like Michelle, you should naturally

Michelle Wie's Power-Swing: Caught on Camera

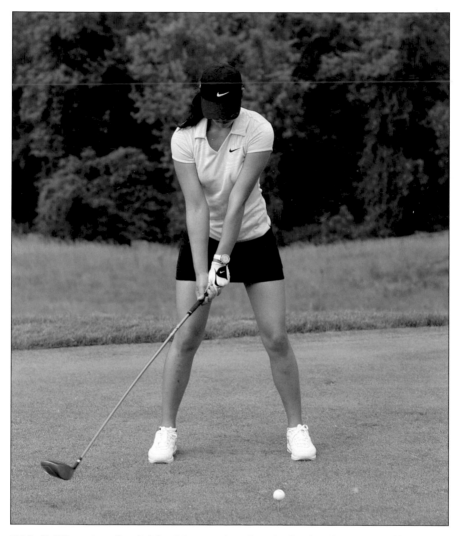

Michelle Wie swings the club back in one piece, keeping her hands, wrists, and lower body passive. This early takeaway action stands in sharp contrast to those employed by many amateur players, who drain power from their swing by hinging their wrists too soon and also turning their hips prematurely on an exaggerated flat plane.

What you cannot see from looking at the photograph above is the smoothness of Michelle's swing tempo in this early stage of the backswing. How important is this?

"With a slower backswing, I actually get more speed coming down," said Wie in the November 2005 issue of *Golf Digest* magazine.

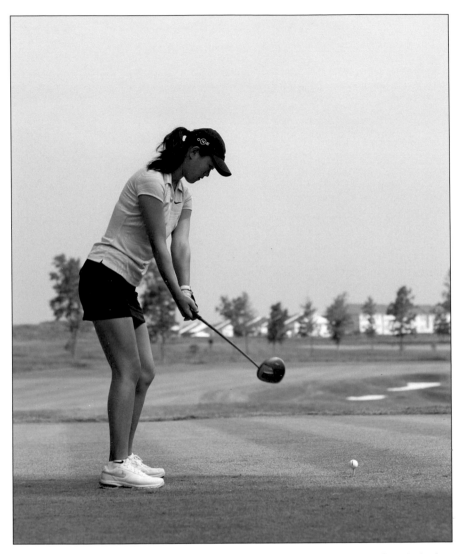

Wie's late takeaway position is absolutely flawless, particularly because the club shaft is extended back in front of her body, helping her create power via a wide swing arc.

In order to match Wie's extended takeaway action, heed this advice from innovative golf instructor Don Trahan, author of the book *Golf, Plain and Simple:*

"Imagine a baseball catcher directly behind your line of flight, with his glove out-stretched.

"Think of the catcher's mitt being held as a target over the low-inside corner of the plate, about two feet behind you and elevated above the ground.

"Up to the point that you have placed the club head in the mitt, you should make no conscious or forceful movement of your hands, wrists, or arms in swinging the club away."

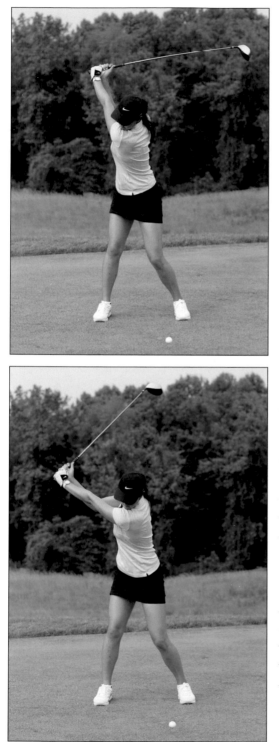

The most exceptional feature of Michelle Wie's backswing involves the way she turns the shoulders far more than the hips, which allows her to create maximum torque in the swing. Wie turns her shoulders 110 degrees, while her hip turn is 45 degrees, illustrated in the photograph shown top left, yielding an X-Factor of 65 degrees:

"The X-Factor is the difference between the degree of shoulder turn and the degree of hip turn when the player is fully coiled at the top of the backswing," said teacher Jim McLean, whom I collaborated with on the book *The X-Factor Swing*.

"The greater the difference between the shoulder and hip turns, the more tension there must be in the player's midsection. This tension reaches its maximum at the very top of the backswing and then is unleashed with the first move into the downswing."

One sure way to promote a strong turn of the shoulders and upper body is to let your head swivel away from the target well before reaching the top of the backswing, as Michelle Wie does in the photograph bottom left.

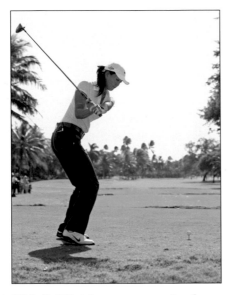

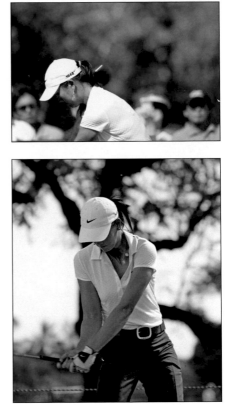

Michelle Wie triggers a more natural downswing by pushing her right hip downward, rotating her right knee inward, and increasing pressure on her right foot almost simultaneously (above, left).

It's this right-sided action that allows the club to drop down from an inside position automatically (above, top right), then return to a position in front of the body with her right wrist still hinged (above, right), but readied to straighten and snap the club powerfully into the ball.

Michelle Wie's right-sided motion is very similar to that of world-renowned power hitter, Mike Dunaway, who told me, "Once you reach to the top of the backswing and feel that your body is ready to spring back toward the target, push your right hip downward, and counterclockwise toward the golf ball and left leg."

That Dunaway is impressed with Wie's swing says something, considering he is a former winner of the World Super Long Drive Contest and has received accolades about his special swing technique from golfing greats, including Ken Venturi, the former U.S. Open champion.

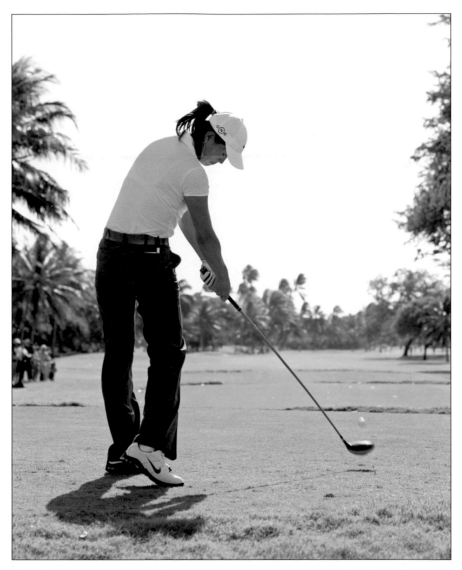

This photograph shows Michelle Wie in the golf swing's moment-of-truth position—impact!

There is no pro golfer today who looks as technically correct in the impact point as Michelle. One chief reason Michelle makes square and solid contact with the ball is that the right side of her lower body hits powerfully against a clearing left hip and braced left leg.

"Leverage, that's Wie's secret," said John Anselmo, the former longtime teacher of Tiger Woods. "Wie's left foot and left leg press down and grab the ground, while her head and upper body stay back — causing her muscles to stretch and the club to gain such speed that it whips hard as it releases powerfully into the ball."

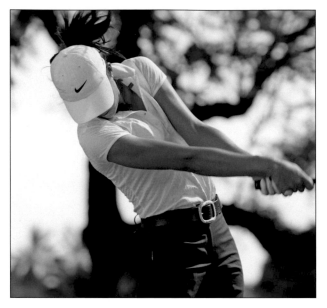

The photograph above shows how Michelle Wie extends her arms in the early follow-through; the photograph below shows how she swings powerfully past impact while maintaining superb balance.

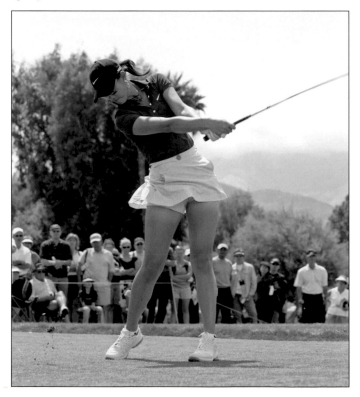

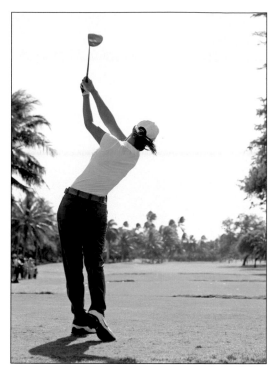

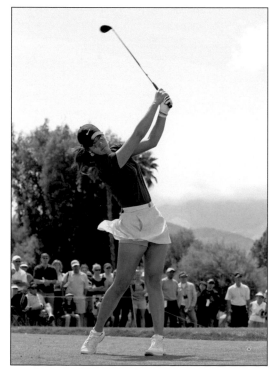

Michelle Wie's late follow-through positions, shown here from two angles, prove that only by swinging at controlled high speed and coordinating the movements of the body with the movements of the club can you employ a fluid release action.

"Michelle's head rotates toward the target and her body releases fully, indicating the tempo, timing, and rhythm of her swing were all in sync," says Gerald Walford, ranked among the top sixty World Golf Teachers Federation teachers.

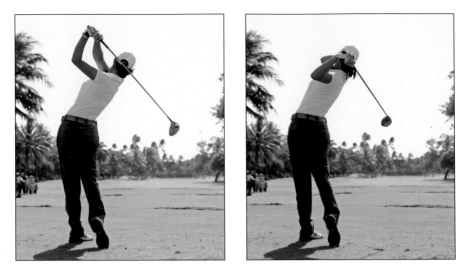

The photographs above, showing Michelle Wie in the early finish position (left) and the late finish (right), remind me of former Masters champion and long hitter Fred Couples, who also looks super-relaxed when completing the swing.

What these positions indicate is that Michelle's grip is pressure free during the address, backswing, and pre-finish position of the downswing. When addressing the ball, average golfers make the mistake of squeezing the club too hard, then upon reaching the top of the swing squeeze even harder as they pull the club into the ball, rather than letting the hands stay relaxed when swinging the club down and through the impact zone.

My advice: Before you swing, let Wie's finish positions play in your mind's eye like two sequential frames in a movie. Conditioning yourself to visualize a finish like Wie's will promote a free-flowing downswing motion critical to accelerating the club through the ball at maximum speed.

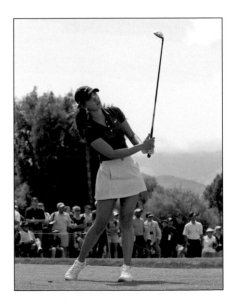

Something else you should do after finishing the swing: let the club recoil back down in front of you, then watch the flight of the ball as Michelle Wie is shown doing in the photograph at right. Analyzing the pattern of the ball's flight (e.g., left to right) and its trajectory (e.g., low), will provide you with instant feedback on your swing's status quo. For example, a low shot hit right of target indicates that you are leaving too much weight on your right side at impact, and arriving at the ball with the club face open.

begin to cock your right arm at the elbow; when you do this, the hinging of your wrists should naturally follow, as it does for Michelle.

Michelle keeps her left arm extended all the way to the top of the backswing. Many golfers do find, however, that as they lift and hinge the right arm, not only will the wrists begin to hinge, but often, the left arm will begin to bend at this point also. Naturally, it is best if only your wrists hinge, albeit minimally, so that your left arm remains firm and the resulting arc of your swing remains as wide as possible. However, it is my observation that some golfers are born with the ability to hinge or cock the wrists more freely than others.

A golfer who does not have as much hinge in the wrists may find that his or her left elbow will start to give or bend somewhat at this point in the backswing, in response to the upward hinging of the right arm. If this is the case with you, it is better that you allow a slight amount of bending to occur in the left arm, because any conscious effort to force your left arm to remain straight does much more harm than good, by destroying the timing and flow of your swing.

Another point that deserves close study here is the position of Michelle's right knee, a major focal point in the teachings of instructor Phil Ritson. Ritson, an early mentor to Wie's present coach, David Leadbetter, is one of the most learned of all golf coaches and a true teaching guru, as I learned in 1992 when collaborating with him on *Golf*

Your Way. I've also taken lessons from Ritson at the Orange County National Golf Center & Lodge in Winter Garden, Florida, and it was during one of our sessions that he explained the vital importance that the right knee plays in the golf swing.

"The right knee is a highly critical link to employing a good backswing and strong upper body turn," said Ritson.

"You must maintain the flex in the right knee when swinging back, so that weight shifts solidly into the right leg and foot.

"There's a tendency on the part of the average golfer to let the right knee buckle outward. This fault triggers excessive lateral upper body and head movement. In turn, this sway causes power to be drained from the swing, via a weak body turn."

I am sure that Leadbetter agrees with Ritson on the importance of the right knee in the golf swing. Having taken lessons at "Lead's" present base, Champions Gate in Davenport, Florida, spoken to him about golf technique when he taught formerly at Lake Nona Golf Club in Orlando, Florida, while I was a member there, and worked with him on instructional pieces for *Golf Magazine*, I can assure you that he also believes the right knee must maintain its flex to create resistance or torque. However, Leadbetter takes things up a notch by wanting the right knee to swivel slightly as the player swings from address to the top, an idea I think is very intelligent and one of Michelle Wie's secrets to looking so free as she employs a very strong turn on the backswing.

The right knee must act as a resistor or a brace against the shifting of the weight to the right that occurs throughout the backswing motion. Miro Bellagamba, the late great golf instructor who was affiliated with the United States Golf Teachers Federation and an individual who seemed to always have the inside scoop on a golf story, told me that before Michelle Wie started working with Leadbetter, she was letting the right knee slide outward. This fault caused her upper body to sway to the right on the backswing and, in turn, hindered her delivery of club-into-ball and her ability to hit good golf shots. I can understand how this fault could happen, knowing that it is not easy or all that natural to hold the right knee in its flexed, yet stable position as it accepts the transfer of a large percentage of the body's weight. It is even possible that as a thirteen-year-old Wie simply was not strong enough in her legs to keep the right knee from buckling outward, and swaying with the upper body.

Michelle's current right knee position, by Leadbetter's or virtually any other highly experienced teacher's definition, is perfect. Michelle maintains a slight flex in the knee, yet the kneecap swivels just a bit to the right as compared to at address, just as Leadbetter has suggested it should.

As a point of comparison, it might prove useful to compare Michelle's position at this stage in the backswing to that of golf's greatest prodigy of a decade ago, Tiger Woods. My book *The Tiger Woods Way* features a sequence of photos of Tiger swinging the driver that was taken in 1996, the year Tiger turned pro at age twenty. I'd like to add here that this might be a point for debate among top instructors, but it is the feeling of many, myself included, that this is the period of time in which Tiger Woods was swinging the golf club the best that he ever has. Mind you, I am not saying that this was when Tiger Woods was the best player he has ever been. In the decade that has passed, he has improved immensely in the areas of short game shots, putting, and overall course management as well as emotional management. His twelve major professional championships are irrefutable proof of major improvement in all these areas. Still, it's very doubtful to me that Tiger Woods swings the golf club any better today than he did in 1996.

That said, if you compare current photos of Michelle and of Tiger in 1996, their swings at the same point three-quarters of the way into the backswing share a great many similarities, but a couple of significant differences. In terms of the amount of shoulder (and torso) turn to this point, the edge goes to Tiger. His shoulders have turned just about 90 degrees, a really amazing amount of turn for this point in the backswing. Michelle, as stated earlier, has turned her shoulders about 75 degrees from their starting point— excellent but not quite a match for Tiger.

However, with regard to the positioning of the right

knee at this point, while both are exceptionally good, it is Michelle who does the slightly better job of bracing the right knee. Her entire right leg, from ankle up to hip, is still angled inward by about 15 degrees, just as it was at address; Tiger's right knee, by comparison, has moved just a little to the right from where it was at address, so that the entire leg is angled in a little less than Michelle's. This observation is not meant to be a criticism of Tiger. I would just say that, with his massive body coil, there had to be a great deal of pressure on Tiger's right knee, so that it did move to the right a little. To put it another way, Tiger's windup was probably a little closer to his personal "redline," the point where he could lose balance and control of his swing arc, than Michelle is to hers at this point in the backswing. Any way you look at it, Michelle has achieved a textbook position at this point in her backswing. Let me remind you, though, this firmly braced right knee is not an easy position to accomplish on the backswing. Michelle had to work hard to perfect her right knee hold-and-swivel action. But hold her right knee position she does, and this adds tremendous stability and power to her backswing.

In order to make a consistent, repeating swing, you too must learn to keep the right knee's position stable throughout the backswing. Practice making your backswing coil in slow motion, using your upper torso to make the turn, and allowing your body weight to shift onto your right leg. If you do this correctly, you should feel some pressure on the inside of your right thigh, just above the knee. Conversely, if you don't feel any pressure, it almost certainly means that your knee is buckling outward, even when you are paying attention to it. Keep making your full torso turn and keep feeling that weight move onto the inside (never the outside) of that right leg. If you have been in the habit of letting your right or rear knee buckle outward, you'll probably need to keep practicing this until the inside of your right leg actually feels fatigued. Keep working at it; gradually you will build up the strength needed to hold the knee in position under the full stress of the backswing turn, just as Michelle Wie did.

Swinging to the Top: Compact and Coiled

From three-quarters of the way through the backswing, Michelle makes a number of marvelous moves that allow her to reach her top-of-backswing position with a tremendous body coil, but with a backswing that is still compact and well under control.

Let's take a close look at the individual bodily movements Michelle makes to get to this position, starting from the ground up. After explaining all of these, and comparing her positions with those of other top players, I will also provide summarizing commentary on her overall position with the driver at the top, so that the instructional messages involving this extremely important area of the swing are clear.

One of the most remarkable points regarding Wie's at-the-top position involves her left foot, which remains virtually dead flat on the ground. There may be a little more pressure on the inside of the left foot than there was at address, but there is no visible turn onto the inside of the left foot; the outside of the left sole does not come off the ground. Nor has Michelle's left heel been pulled off the ground by her torso turn. If you were to compare Michelle's left foot position at the top with that of Jack Nicklaus in his prime, you would see a tremendous contrast. When Nicklaus employed a full driver swing, his huge torso-and-hip turn pulled his weight to the inside of the left foot, so that the outside of the left sole was slightly off the ground, and the left heel of his golf shoe was pulled about one full inch off the ground.

You might quite reasonably ask, "Should I let my left heel rise off the ground or not?" The answer to this question: Neither method is actually 100 percent correct or 100 percent incorrect. The contrasting left foot/heel positions of Wie and Nicklaus are merely indicative of the differences in flexibility of Wie as opposed to Nicklaus in his prime. As we know of Nicklaus and as we see with Wie, both make extremely full body turns on the backswing. The difference is that Michelle is able to maximize her turn while keeping her left foot flat on the ground, because she is much more flexible than Nicklaus was during his heyday of the 1960s. In order to maximize his turn, Nicklaus had to allow his left heel to rise. If he had made a conscious effort to keep his left foot flat, his torso and hip turns would have been much more limited. As a result, he would not have been able to produce nearly the amount of pent-up power at the top of his backswing, as he did by allowing his left heel to lift.

Michelle Wie, on the other hand, can generate a remarkably full body turn without allowing her left heel to rise, because of her flexibility. It is a definite advantage that Michelle is able to accomplish this, because keeping the left foot flat can only lead to greater overall consistency. You might say that Michelle has one less moving part.

The observant student might ask, "Shouldn't Michelle, like Nicklaus, make an even bigger backswing coil, to the point where even her left heel gets pulled from the ground, in order to create even greater power than she does already on the backswing and to ultimately help her hit the ball even longer?"

Yes, Michelle Wie certainly could try for an even bigger coil. But with that attempt she would run the risk of over-swinging in a number of different ways; not only in terms of making the club shaft dip far below parallel at the top, à la John Daly, but also of possibly losing that great right knee brace that we have talked about, and swaying off the ball to the right. At present, Michelle makes the largest possible coil while keeping the left foot in one spot. In doing so, she achieves the best of both worlds—a very powerful coil that is also very much under control. Therefore, the answer to that question is *no*.

Another feature of Michelle Wie's backswing that I find interesting and technically enlightening involves the change in the position of her left knee. Throughout the backswing motion, the left knee is gradually pulled inward, or to the right, by perhaps four inches from its position at address. Her left kneecap, which was just in front of the ball's position at the start, rotates just behind it as she continues swinging back. Make sure you understand: Wie makes no conscious effort to move the left knee inward, and neither should you. Her left knee movement is merely part of a chain reaction; the tremendous clockwise coiling of her upper torso forces her hips to turn in the same direction, which in turn forces the knee inward. However, her coil does not, as we've just discussed, force her left foot to roll inward or her left heel to lift.

If you are a golfer with average flexibility, your left or forward knee should definitely rotate inward by several inches as you make your upper body coil. If you were to try to hold that knee in place throughout the swing, one of two negative things would likely be bound to happen:

1. You make a very limited body turn, thus greatly reducing the amount of pent-up power at the top of the backswing.

2. You keep most of your weight on your left or forward foot as you reach the top, so that a reverse pivot on the downswing, in which your weight would fall back to the right, is inevitable.

Your Lesson

Let the left knee swivel inward naturally. You may very well find that you will also have to allow the weight on your left leg to roll to the inside of your left foot, and/or allow your left heel to rise, in order to complete a good full turn. If so, that's what you should do, especially if you want to get the utmost power out of your golf swing.

Next, let's look at Michelle's hip turn. While it is obvious that the hips have turned, they have not turned an extreme amount—perhaps 45 degrees from their starting position. (As a point of comparison, John Daly, who makes perhaps the biggest hip turn as well as shoulder turn in the game, has had his hip turn measured at 66 degrees with the driver.) What Michelle's amount of hip turn tells us is that her hips, too, are turning in response to the turning of her upper torso—they are being pulled along for the ride. Wie does not make a conscious effort to turn her hips as far as she can. (We will talk much more about this point, both as it regards Wie and how it applies to your own game, in a moment.)

Now let's move up to observe Michelle's shoulder turn. It is massive: She turns her shoulders approximately 110

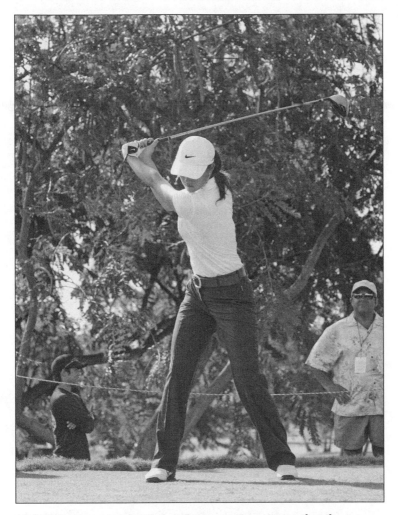

Michelle's compact and coiled at-the-top position proves that the backswing does not have to be long to create power. The secret to building torque in the swing revolves around the relationship between the degree of shoulder turn and hip turn.

It's also important to note that ever since shortening her backswing under the guidance of David Leadbetter and his associate Gary Gilchrist, Michelle has gained added control on her drives.

degrees from their original position. Few golfers, professional or amateur, can muster this degree of shoulder turn under any circumstances, but definitely not while maintaining the lower-body stability that Michelle exhibits. By comparison, Tiger Woods, at age twenty, turned his shoulders approximately 100 degrees from the address position, perhaps just a shade more. It is true that John Daly, probably the longest hitter in the game over the entirety of the last fifteen years, has had a shoulder turn measured at some 120 degrees. However, as I mentioned already, Daly also makes a conscious, huge hip turn. In doing so, the lower half of his body is providing less resistance to the coiling of his upper body, when compared to Wie's action. This brings us to an opportune point at which to digress slightly and consider a factor in the backswing that is a key producer of power.

The Secret to Distance: The X-Factor

We have talked about Michelle Wie's tremendous shoulder turn, and what some might think of as a moderate amount of hip turn. "Isn't it desirable," you might ask, "to have the largest possible amounts of both shoulder and hip turn, while still keeping the body and the club under control?"

In answering this logical question, I would like to reiterate some relevant points about the backswing related to me by noted teacher Jim McLean, with whom I collaborated on an instruction book titled *The X-Factor Swing*. In the early 1990s, McLean along with Mike McTeigue (a golf pro who invented a swing measuring apparatus known as the SportSense Motion Trainer), measured both the hip and shoulder turns of countless players, most notably top PGA Tour professionals.

"The majority of amateur players who visit my schools or I speak to while on the road think they should turn their shoulders and their hips as much as they can on the backswing and that the harder they swing at the ball the farther the ball will fly," said McLean.

"After testing many top Tour pros, I helped disprove this widely accepted fundamental of the swing—that to generate maximum power the golfer should turn the hips and shoulders to the max.

"What I and Mike McTeigue discovered was this: The generation of high club-head speed and power in the golf swing has a direct relationship to the creation of a gap, or differential, between the shoulder and hip turn. In general, the bigger the differential, the farther you hit the ball."

The X-Factor, then, is the difference between the degree of shoulder turn and the degree of hip turn when the player is fully coiled at the top of the backswing. The greater the difference between shoulder- and hip-turns, the more tension there must be in the player's midsection—the area between the hips and the shoulders that is being both stretched and twisted by the action of the backswing. This tension reaches its maximum at the very top of the backswing, and then is unleashed with the first move into the downswing (the subject of the next chapter).

In Michelle Wie's case, her extremely full shoulder turn is 110 degrees, and her hip turn is some 45 degrees (remember, her hips turn only as far as they must, in response to the pull of the shoulder turn). When you do the math, Wie's backswing has an X-Factor of 65 degrees (110-degree shoulder turn minus 45-degree hip turn). Although it cannot be stated with certainty, because most players, even on the PGA Tour, have not been measured for this differential, the evidence that exists shows that Michelle Wie's current swing exhibits the highest X-Factor rating in golf. For points of comparison, Tiger Woods' driver swing of 1996 displayed an X-Factor of about 55 degrees (100-degree shoulder turn minus 45-degree hip turn). If anything, Woods' X-Factor reading might be a shade lower at age thirty than it was at age twenty (due to a slightly smaller shoulder turn). John Daly, meanwhile, has a massive 120-degree shoulder turn with his driver, but also a massive hip turn (measured at 66 degrees). This gives him an X-Factor of 54, a substantial number, but less than Woods' reading and substantially lower than Wie's.

Keep in mind, the X-Factor is definitely not the only factor that determines how far Michelle Wie, or you, or any other golfer, can hit your drives. Overall height and weight, agility, strength in the hands and arms, body flexibility, hand-eye coordination, and numerous other factors come into the equation. However, the X-Factor theory goes a long way to explaining how Michelle Wie, even at a very slender 145 pounds, is able to bomb tee shots that most male amateurs can only dream of. Under Leadbetter's tutelage, she has learned to build a tremendous amount of power-producing tension in her golf swing, yet at the same time, make a swing that is wonderfully under control.

It's unlikely that you will be able to employ the exact same backswing as Wie, yet you can increase your X-Factor by starting a program to strengthen your abdominal muscles. You can do this in a relatively short period of time, either at a gym or in your own home. This is one of the best-kept secrets to building a more powerful golf swing and a program Jim Hardy recommends to his amateur and pro golf students.

You can condition your abdominals without using any weights at all, simply by doing several sets of sit-ups every day. Even better than sit-ups are crunches—simply lifting your head and shoulders straight up off the floor by just a couple of inches from a normal sit-up position lying on the floor. You can make these crunches more challenging by doing them while holding a hand weight in each of your hands, with each positioned on either side of your head. Also, you can perform windmills, which will stretch and strengthen the muscles of your sides. Stand up and spread your arms out at full length to either side. Next, simply twist your abdomen in one direction then the other, repeatedly. If you perform just these two exercises every day for a few weeks, you will probably start to feel and see the difference in your backswing coil out on the course.

Naturally, if you have access to a fitness center, there are a number of easy-to-use machines that will stretch and strengthen your abdominal muscles, allowing you to see results even more quickly. Now, having examined Michelle's top-of-backswing position from the feet through the shoulders, and explained the source of her pent-up power to this point in the swing, let's continue by studying what Michelle does from the shoulders up.

Probably the most important point here is the positioning of Michelle's head. Back at the address, while her head was stationed behind the ball, her chin was pointing slightly forward, right at the golf ball. However, as Michelle reaches the top, she allows her head to swivel to the right. Note that I said her head "swivels" to the right rather than moves laterally to the right. Michelle doesn't move her head from its relative position in space, but it is very evident that her head swivels, so that her chin points well to the outside, or to the right of, her right foot. This is a really extensive swivel, and most of it occurs from the time her club shaft is three-quarters of the way back (i.e., pointing straight up), until the very top of the backswing. This is something that Michelle, or any player who makes a big shoulder turn, has to do in order to prevent the chin from blocking the clockwise movement of the left shoulder. I doubt that anyone

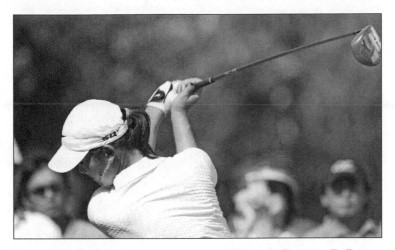

Letting your head swivel on the backswing, like Michelle Wie, will allow you to "max out" your shoulder turn and increase your personal X-Factor.

taught Michelle to swivel her head as she does. Rather, it is an intuitive reaction that allows her to complete her backswing without knocking herself out of balance.

This particular facet of Wie's backswing is quite fascinating, especially in light of the fact that most golfers, from the first day they hold a club, are instructed to "keep the head still" from the start of the swing to its finish. Some golfers try so hard to keep their heads stock-still that they minimize or cut off their own backswing turns. Not only does this greatly reduce their power, but it also badly disrupts any sense of timing in the swing.

You will be far better off regarding how still you keep your head by following the example of Wie or one of the most powerful players (as well as the greatest) of his era,

Jack Nicklaus. The Golden Bear also swiveled his head to the right to make space for his shoulder turn. The difference between Nicklaus and Wie is that Jack made a conscious swiveling move to the right with his head, as a triggering move just before he started the backswing. Wie does it more instinctively as her shoulders approach the completion of their turn. If you compare Nicklaus' early head movement with Wie's, though, you'll note they have an almost identical amount of head swivel. All in all, then, it is good advice for any golfer, but especially for those of you seeking to lengthen your drives, to allow the head to swivel rather than restricting your backswing turn by fighting to keep your head perfectly still.

Hands High, but Also Deep

The next technical point to appreciate is how high Michelle's hands are at the top of the backswing. Michelle's hands are a good six inches above the top of her head, obviously maintaining a tremendously wide arc at the top. Her high hand position is very reminiscent of that of PGA Tour player and former PGA champion Davis Love III, who is still one of the game's longest hitters.

In spite of her high hands, it is very pertinent to note that Michelle's arm swing is only moderately upright. When viewed from behind, it's easy to see that Michelle's left arm is swinging on a plane that is about 50 degrees up from horizontal. Furthermore, if you were to draw a line along the plane of her left arm at the top of the backswing, it would point just outside the ball. This is a good checkpoint for higher-handicap amateurs, particularly taller ones who often swing their arms on an exaggerated upright plane or angle. Many people have the misconception that a swing that is very upright is better than a flatter one, based on the reasoning that if the path of the club head stays closer to the target line throughout the swing, the chances are better that the club face will be square to the target line at impact.

While it's true that the path of the club stays closer to the target line with a more upright arm swing, keep in mind that this does not mean that it is easier for the club face itself to get back to perfectly square at impact. In fact, it is actually a little harder to deliver the face squarely to the ball. There's no point in getting into great technical detail here, but suffice it to say that the more upright the swing, the faster the club face must move from a very open position shortly before impact, to square at impact, and then to a very closed position just after impact. These complex movements of the club require perfect timing of a very fast rotation of the forearms in a counterclockwise direction. That's a lot to ask of any golfer, even as talented a player as Michelle Wie.

A second problem that occurs when the arm swing (and thus the club head's path) is too upright is that the club head will be entering the impact zone on a steep angle, that is, from too much above the ball. Thus the player will be delivering a downward blow. This is not all bad when the player is hitting a short iron or one of the wedges. However, it robs the player of a great deal of distance with the driver; with this club and a teed-up ball, it's imperative to deliver the club levelly in the hitting area, in order to give the ball maximum forward thrust (as opposed to swinging sharply downward and imparting exaggerated backspin on the ball). All that said, Michelle's arm-swing angle has brought the driver up on an excellent plane, with her hands positioned fairly deep behind her head, rather than being more directly above it.

Shoulders Turn Flatter

Despite the fact that Michelle's arm swing is only moderately upright, the plane formed by her left arm, which we estimated at 50 degrees up from horizontal, is still much more upright than the plane on which she turns her shoulders. If you recall, we noted earlier that at address, Michelle's spine was tilted forward at about 25 degrees below perpendicular. At the top of the backswing, Michelle's shoulders have turned around her spine at about that same 25-degree angle. She does not tilt her shoulders in relation to the angle of her spine; she does not allow the left shoulder to dip on the backswing while the right shoulder rises up. If anything, Michelle's shoulders turn on an angle that is perhaps a degree or two shallower than they were set on at address. This would indicate that, if anything, Michelle's spine angle has lifted just a touch from the position that she started in. This is a very minor flaw, and is also one of the reasons Michelle can create such a wide arc. If she were to lower her spine angle during the backswing, that would be a greater cause for concern, as this would narrow her arc and reduce her power.

Be that as it may, there is a noticeable gap or an angle between Wie's left arm swing, and the angle of her shoulder turn, which is approximately 25 degrees. This is the result of the natural lifting motion that is added by the folding of the right arm during the second half of the backswing, which we have already discussed. Such a gap is quite common; in fact, the angle between arm swing and shoulder turn is often much larger.

In *The Plane Truth for Golfers*, a book I collaborated on in 2005, veteran teacher Jim Hardy expounds on his theory that there are two types of swings: a one-plane swing in which the shoulders and the arms move along a single plane line through the backswing and downswing; and a two-plane swing, in which the shoulders turn on a relatively shallow plane, while the arms swing on a more upright one. Hardy cited Wie as a "pure one-planer."

Based on Jim Hardy's definition, Michelle Wie's top-of-backswing position clearly indicates to me that she *now* employs a two-plane golf swing. There is nothing wrong with

Wie making a change, considering that even Hardy makes it clear that both swings can work very successfully. Besides, I believe one person in particular—John Jacobs, the great British teacher who exerted a tremendous influence on many instructors, including Hardy—would be pleased with Wie's choice, extrapolating from Jacobs' assertion in his book *Practical Golf*: "If the arms are to position the club correctly in the backswing, and swing freely in the through swing, they must swing up as the shoulders turn around."

When Michelle Wie swings back to the top, the fact that her left arm swings at some 25 degrees higher than the angle of her shoulder turn necessitates that she make an equal amount of downward motion with her arms to deliver the club face squarely and solidly into the ball. However, as you'll soon learn, she's able to do that nine out of ten times. This is one chief reason why I think Michelle should continue on a two-plane swinger. Here are my other reasons:

First, Wie has exhibited a tremendous combination of power and accuracy with her current swing. She has the capability of becoming the finest ball striker among women players that the game has seen. Any major change to her current action would, I believe, be extremely risky on her part.

Second, it should be noted that the action that causes the primary difference between the one- and two-plane swings—that is, the lifting of the arms during the backswing and their downward drive on the downswing—is a significant source of power in any two-plane swing. Another way of putting it: While the one-plane swing may, at least theoretically, provide greater consistency, the two-plane swing almost certainly has the advantage of developing greater power. And it is the power in Michelle Wie's golf swing that makes her likely to set a new level for what the woman golfer can achieve, at least in terms of the full swing.

Finally, I would add that although Michelle's swing would fall into the two-plane category, it is what I would call a very moderate two-plane swing. The difference in the angles at which she swings her arms and turns her shoulders is relatively small. True, if she were to swing her arms straight up while turning her shoulders horizontally, it would undoubtedly be a very ungainly, hard-to-control action. However, this theory of the two-plane swing is really a matter of degrees, if you will. Michelle Wie has a two-plane golf swing, but, again, it is a very moderate two-plane golf swing. As such, the odds are extremely good that it will stand up to the test of time.

Left Wrist Stays Flat

One of the reasons that Michelle Wie is such a consistent as well as powerful striker of the ball is that she maintains a straight or "flat" left wrist throughout the backswing, and maintains this flat position as she sets the club at the top.

The back of her left hand, the wrist itself, and her left arm all remain flat in a straight line, virtually the same as they were at address.

The flat left wrist position is one golf instructor John Anselmo stressed Tiger Woods adopt and check constantly when teaching him from the ages of ten through seventeen. According to Anselmo, a flat left wrist position on the backswing helps the golfer maintain a square club-face position at impact and hit accurate shots, whereas either a cupped or bowed position at the top of the backswing requires that the golfer steer the club into impact, which in turn can cause the golfer to hit off-line shots of sundry shapes and trajectories.

Another key technical point in Michelle's backswing worth noting: The driver's club face lies on precisely the same plane as a line drawn along her left arm. If the back of Michelle's left wrist were bowed at the top, the club face would be pointing very closed, or more toward the sky. If her left wrist were cupped inward (and this is probably the more common error of the two) the club face would be very open, with the toe pointing more directly at the ground. Either fault would require a correction of the left wrist angle, and with it, the club face during the downswing. Any such correction in the split second it takes to execute the downswing is a dicey proposition at best.

If you are not sure if you've arrived at the top of the swing with your left wrist flat (and your right wrist bent back), ask a friend to analyze your backswing on the practice tee. (*Note*: Ask him or her to check your action while you are hitting actual shots. Even though it is harder to judge during a "real" swing, you will get a truer reading from the swing you make on actual shots than you would by posing in the at-the-top backswing position.) If your left wrist isn't flat at the top and you are not sure how to get it there, heed the advice of David Leadbetter and many other top instructors who encourage students to feel that the left thumb supports the club shaft. If your left thumb is not supporting the shaft from directly underneath it, the wrist is likely to bend one way or the other. Although it is difficult to pick up in photographs because the left thumb is underneath the base of the right thumb, you can readily see from a face-on view of Wie's top-of-backswing position that her left thumb is directly underneath the shaft.

Right Arm L- and Tray-Positions

A final element of Michelle's top-of-backswing that I find very admirable is the position of her right arm. Her right forearm and the upper part of her right arm are essentially at right angles to one another and form the letter L. Michelle's right forearm is thus in the ideal position to support the weight of the club when she swings back to the top.

One way to groove this L-position is to practice a drill taught at the David Leadbetter Golf Academy at Champions Gate in Davenport, Florida. Here's how it works:

Step 1: Hold a medium iron in your right hand only.

Step 2: Take your address.

Step 3: Swing the club to the top, allowing your right arm to hinge at the elbow quite early in the takeaway.

Step 4: Stop and feel the vital L-position.

Step 5: Once you understand the motion physically and have a vivid mental image of the L-position formed in your mind's eye, tee up a few balls and actually hit shots.

Step 6: Note how your new backswing move helps your downswing flow more fluidly.

Step 7: Take out your driver and hit a few tee shots. (You'll be shocked, as I was, by how far and straight you hit the ball.)

Because Michelle's right elbow is also positioned well out away from her body, some swing purists criticize this as being a "flying right elbow," a somewhat vaguely described element of the top-of-backswing position that, according to many top teachers, should be avoided at all cost.

I disagree, and not just because Jack Nicklaus played great golf for a long time with a flying right elbow or that John Daly and Fred Couples also make it work for them. If

Michelle were to try to keep her right elbow tucked in close to her right side, as is often advised by golf instructors, her swing would be much flatter and the width of her arc far narrower, resulting in a much less powerful action. So, don't be too concerned about whether your elbow is flying or not. If you can achieve what masterful golf instructor Phil Ritson coined the "waiter's tray" position at the top of your backswing—with your right or rear forearm directly underneath and supporting an imaginary tray—you will also be supporting the club well, while at the same time developing a wide, powerful arc for the swinging club head.

Let's sum up the instructional message relayed to you in this chapter. Michelle Wie has reached the top of her backswing by fully coiling or loading the large upper body muscles over her right knee. There is tremendous tension in her upper right leg. She has braced that leg against her upper body coil in order to maintain a stable position, rather than swaying off the ball. She has swiveled her head well to the right as the backswing has progressed, in order to allow room to complete her massive shoulder turn. Her body has turned around her spine, with no added tilting of the shoulders, while her arms have swung on a slightly more upright plane, which gets the hands high at the top and adds power to that which she generates with her body turn.

Michelle Wie is in the ideal position at the top of the backswing to unleash the club on the downswing. In the next section, we will examine precisely how she does that.

MICHELLE WIE'S MASTERFUL BACKSWING POSITIONS

Michelle's hands and the club move back from the ball in response to the turn of her torso, rather than starting back independently. Following Michelle's example will smooth out the tempo, timing, and rhythm of your swing.

Michelle extends her hands, arms, and the golf club back a long way in the takeaway, while keeping her wrists locked. Her one-piece coordinated move will help you create the widest possible arc of backswing and hit longer drives.

Michelle keeps her right knee firmly braced during the backswing—with the inside of that leg holding her weight over the ball—as opposed to letting it sag or sway off the ball or to the right.

Keeping your right knee braced will help you reduce your hip turn and increase your backswing's X-Factor, and that's vital to adding power to your shots.

Michelle's shoulder turn on the backswing is 110 degrees, while the hips coil only 45 degrees.

Following Michelle's example of coiling the upper body against a restricting lower body will help you create powerful torque that at impact will translate to higher club-head speed.

Michelle's left wrist is flat at the top of the backswing (there is no indentation in the wrist area, between the back of the left hand and the top of the left forearm).

Arriving in the same position as Michelle at the top, with your left wrist flat and square to the club face, will help you hit controlled power shots off the tee.

POW!

Michelle Wie's wonderful way of rhythmically coordinating the movement of the body with the movement of the club, as well as the manner in which she contacts the ball solidly on the upswing, are features of her swing well worth copying

Michelle Wie has reached the top of her wide, well-coiled, and majestic top-of-backswing position. What happens next in her process of delivering all this power to that teed-up ball?

There are three popular theories among golf's top teachers about what happens to complete the backswing and start the downswing:

1. There is an overlap of the movements in the two halves of the swing. As the player has just about but not quite finished turning his or her upper body, while the hands and the club have not quite reached their highest point in the backswing, the player actually starts the downswing

by shifting the hips laterally toward the target. This lateral move of the hips puts so much stress on the coil of the upper body that it is automatically forced to begin uncoiling, like a taut rubber band whose tension is released, snapping the band back. (I disagree with this "movement-in-two-directions-at-the-completion-of-the-backswing" concept. I do not think it is even possible for any golfer to consciously, and successfully, make a lateral move with the hips toward the target, while the hands and the club are still ascending to the top of the backswing. There is simply too much happening in too short a time to execute this move, for the amateur player in particular.)

2. The player winds the hips and shoulders so far around in a clockwise direction that the force of the windup catapults the arms, body, and club down, due to centrifugal force. In other words, the downswing is triggered automatically. (Although I agree that centrifugal force plays a key role in the downswing, by virtue of the arms and club swinging outward from the body's center toward the ball, I don't agree with the theory that the downswing just happens by some form of Houdini-like magical spring-back action. On the contrary, it must be triggered by a specific move.)

3. The theory of synchronization calls for the player first to start the backswing by rotating the left knee inward, turning the left shoulder under the chin, coiling the left hip clockwise, and pushing the club away with the left

hand on the backswing. Second, to trigger the downswing action by doing the opposite—simultaneously turning the left knee outward toward the target, rotating the left shoulder up and away from the chin, uncoiling the left hip in a counterclockwise direction, and pulling the club down with the left hand. (I disagree with this theory on the basis that it is unnatural for a right-handed player to employ left-hand triggers. In fact, you'll soon be hearing more on this subject.)

I've just cited the three main theories, but in fact, the list goes on; it's so exhaustive that you can appreciate that when the subjects of completing the backswing and making the transition into the downswing come up among golf instructors, an air of absurdity definitely overwhelms the room.

I'm not sure whether it's a question of the typical teacher wanting to be different than his or her fellow instructors in order to drum up new business, or that teachers are confused themselves by the various articles they read in golf magazines, not to mention the sundry swing theories put forth by golf instructors at local clinics, at the annual PGA Teaching Summit, or on The Golf Channel's nightly *Academy Live* show. Whatever the reason, if teachers themselves are puzzled about downswing triggers, it's no wonder that you and other golfers across America are befuddled.

Before I go any further, I want to make a couple of things clear about the golf swing.

After a golfer swings the club back from the static address position to the top (a segment of the swing that takes on average one and one-half seconds), the body and club do pause, albeit for only a moment, before transitioning into the downswing action. Furthermore, in total, it takes only one-fifth of a second for the average golfer to swing the club down from the top into the ball. Consequently, the player does not realistically have any time to mentally connect the dots in order to consciously direct the downward action of the golf club into the ball. All the same, a physical trigger is required by the golfer to trigger a chain reaction: a downward domino effect of sorts that allows the arms, body, and club to work in unison, essentially on autopilot. Yet that physical trigger must be well rehearsed through regular practice, because there is no time to think about it when swinging on the golf course. Moreover, this trigger must be the right one technically for you or any other golfer to repeat it over and over and consistently hit good drives.

Average golfers commonly make the mistake of thinking consciously about hitting at the ball, rather than merely swinging through the ball. The sure signs of such a problem: an overly steep downswing plane and pop-up type drives; swiping across the ball with the driver and hitting pull slice shots; keeping the head down and eyes glued to the ball through impact, which results in loss of club-head speed and weak fat shots; a spinning-out action of the left foot, left leg, and left hip that very often causes the golfer to contact the top half of the ball and hit shots well left of target or miss the ball completely!

Whereas most of the problems just cited match up with an overly quick tempo, sometimes in the process of thinking too much about hitting the ball rather than swinging the club at maximum controlled speed, the golfer actually swings too slowly. Long hitter John Daly was the first golfer to bring this to my attention when we worked on the book *Grip It and Rip It!* in 1992.

"As a worldwide golf traveler, I see many amateur golfers, who, for one reason or another, just do not seem to be aggressive through the ball," said Daly.

"Have you ever noticed players like these? They look like pros as they analyze the shot, set up to the ball, and make a beautiful, flowing backswing. Then, I don't know why this happens, but they seem to try to push or steer the club head through the impact zone, rather than use the good turn they've made and freewheel through the point of impact, so they not only lose distance but hit the ball wildly, too."

It is indeed frustrating to see a golfer set up and swing the club back correctly on the proper path and plane, and then mess up things on the downswing. Yet in my understanding, this problem—common to middle- and high-handicap players—can be traced to being brainwashed into believing it should be the left side that controls the downswing.

When golf started being played in Scotland around six hundred years ago and officially in America around 1888, firsthand accounts by sportswriters and champion players who put down their thoughts in books prove that golfers once depended on the right side to control the swinging action. It was not until the early 1930s, when steel club shafts started replacing hickory shafts and legendary player Byron Nelson popularized what was called the Modern Swing, that professional golf teachers got on this kick about left-sided golf. The ironic tragedy: Ever since that time, average golfers have not really improved at all, with millions of players actually going backwards on the score-improvement curve. That's because it is far less natural to control the downswing with the left side instead of the right side unless you are a left-handed player, and only about 2 percent of the 27 million golfers in the United States swing from the "South Side."

I literally can count on one hand the number of teachers, tour professionals, and television swing analysts who ever mention the importance of the right side controlling the downswing. This is a grave mistake; certainly, if you believe what Spanish golfer and five-time major championship winner Severiano Ballesteros told me when we were collaborating on the instruction book *Natural Golf*:

Because most of the human race is right-handed, left-sided moves very rarely come naturally for most people.

I don't care what many teachers say about golf being a game of opposites. Any time you ask an individual to do something that doesn't click with his nature, it is bound to be both physically difficult and mentally confusing for him or her.

If you're right-handed, I'm convinced you will play golf more easily, and come closer to your ultimate potential, with the emphasis more on your right side than your left side.

Incidentally, "Seve" uttered those words after winning the 1979 British Open, 1980 Masters, 1983 Masters, 1984 British Open, and the 1988 British Open, at a time when he was hitting the ball solidly off the tee, looking free as a bird on the downswing. It was only after he stopped being a self-taught right-sided golfer and started taking lessons from a tour professional and a teacher who both stressed left-sided golf (and whose anonymity I shall respect) that his driving game deteriorated and really never recovered.

Another great player from the past, Curtis Strange, who won the 1988 U.S. Open at The Country Club in Brook-line, Massachusetts, and the 1989 U.S. Open played at Oak Hill Country Club in Rochester, New York, employed a right-sided swing that he learned from Jimmy Ballard, one of the most highly respected golf instructors in the game. The technique allowed Strange to hit solid, super-accurate drives. Ballard, who I remember working with on instructional articles during my tenure at *Golf Magazine*, had this to say in his book *How to Perfect Your Golf Swing*:

In the golf swing, when you achieve a coiled position behind the ball at the top of the backswing, the kick of the right foot and right knee begins a connected chain reaction that is transmitted from the ground up, through your body center and on out through arms, hands, and club.

Of two things I am absolutely certain: (1) There has never been a great striker of the ball who didn't tear at it with the right side, and (2) The right side is the most valuable untapped resource that the average golfer possesses.

I don't know what possessed Curtis to leave Ballard and start messing around with his natural, very rhythmic, easy-to-repeat golf swing. However, I do know this, based on conversations I had with Curtis when I played two rounds of golf with him in Williamsburg, Virginia: He regrets switching teachers and switching from a right-sided to left-sided golf swing.

The biggest reason golfers are failing to take advantage of the great advancements in golf club technology is that they focus too much on the left side, using one of a number of the wrong type triggers. Even Tiger Woods is starting to miss a lot of fairways with the driver because, consciously or unconsciously, he often triggers the downswing with an exaggerated "bump" of the left hip or clears his left hip too early.

Conversely, one chief reason why Michelle Wie continues to hit the ball so solidly down the fairway is that, just after the club stalls for a moment at the top of the backswing (in preparation for the change in direction), she triggers the downswing with the right side of her body.

Before covering the fine points of Michelle Wie's downswing action, let's step back and review her model at-the-top position, so you will be poised to spark the downswing by matching her unique triggers.

At the top of the backswing, Michelle's shoulders and upper torso are wound up fully, with the shoulders turned 110 degrees around from where they started at address. Michelle also turns over a braced right leg position, with no sway to the right; the pressure of her weight is on the inside of her right thigh. Michelle's left arm is extended, too, maximizing the width of her swing arc. Michelle's right elbow is well away from the right side of her body; her right forearm and upper right arm form a right angle, with the forearm pointing straight up and supporting the club's shaft.

One more vital element of Michelle's at-the-top position involves the position of the club: its shaft is parallel to the target line; its face is in a neutral position—neither open nor closed.

Now that you are set at the top, let me discuss Michelle's downswing keys.

I believe Michelle's downswing is triggered by a simultaneous right-sided movement, involving downward pressure put on the right foot, a downward push with the right hip, and an inward rotation of the right knee. Speaking from my experience as a former senior instruction editor at *Golf Magazine*, in which I have probably looked at more sequence swings than just about any PGA instructor, I can say with authority that Wie's three-prong downswing is the most coordinated and best in all of golf. It should also mean something to repeat what Michelle said about her swing in a 2005 issue of *Golf Digest* magazine: "I feel like everything gets to the top together and starts down together."

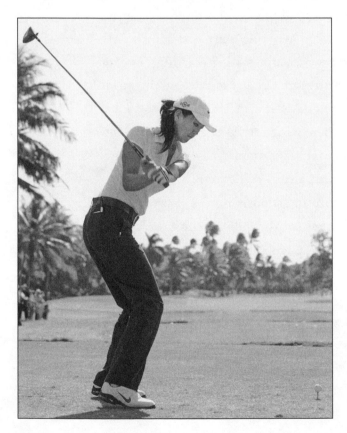

Michelle Wie's natural-feeling three-prong right-sided downswing trigger involves the simultaneous actions of the right foot, right hip, and right knee.

Even though it only takes Wie around one-fifth of a second to swing down into impact from the top of her backswing, here's what occurs once she triggers the downward motion with her right side:

1. Michelle's right hip begins rotating in a counterclockwise direction.
2. Michelle's left knee starts rotating toward the target.
3. Michelle's hands and arms fall freely downward, while the club drops down into a slightly shallower swing plane.
4. Michelle's left knee rotates further inward, so that by the time her hands reach a point level with her chest both knees are braced and square to the target line.
5. Michelle's hips begin shifting laterally.
6. Michelle's arms, hands, and the club drop further downward, with the right elbow and right wrist still hinged.
7. Michelle gets a boost off her right foot as it begins to lift off the ground.
8. Michelle's weight starts shifting quite dramatically to her left foot and stable left leg axis point.
9. Michelle's right shoulder moves down while her left shoulder moves upward.
10. Michelle's left hip rotates briskly in a counterclockwise direction, opening up a clear passageway for the hands and arms to swing the club toward the ball from inside the target line.

11. Michelle's lower body thrust pulls her right foot farther off the ground as more weight shifts to her left foot and braced left leg.

12. Michelle's left arm swings freely and accelerates forward, while her right arm makes a sidearm motion, similar to the one a shortstop employs when throwing a ball to first base, and the right elbow begins straightening.

13. Michelle's upper body and head fall back, away from the target, as the left hip clears and right hip moves more vigorously in a counterclockwise direction.

14. Michelle's hand-arm-club speed increases due to the resistance between an active lower body and passive upper body.

15. Michelle's right wrist starts to unhinge, due to centrifugal force working on the club head.

16. Michelle's left hand really starts rotating and squaring itself to the target, with the club face following suit.

17. Michelle's left leg absorbs her lower body weight and, in bracing, provides her with a firm axis to rotate her hips around and hit powerfully against.

18. Michelle's right hip "fires" fully, causing more of her right foot to come off the ground and give her swing a surge of added power.

19. Michelle enters the impact zone, with stored energy being sent directly into the club head, via her right arm, right wrist, and right hand.

20. Michelle arrives at impact, with her left arm and the club shaft aligned, the majority of her weight on her left foot and leg, all but the front portion of her right foot off the ground, her right elbow and right wrist unhinged fully, the back of her left hand and the palm of her right hand dead square to the target, and the sweet spot of her Nike driver hitting the back center portion of the Nike ball she plays golf with.

21. Michelle hits the ball squarely and solidly. Pow!

One of the most important aspects of the downswing sequence just described is to return the right and left knee into a position similar to what they were in at address, or as Leadbetter puts it in *The Golf Swing*: "The transition from backswing to downswing produces a separation of the knees and a squat, sitting down look in the lower body."

This bracing action of the knees, employed by some legendary drivers of the ball, most notably Sam Snead, Mickey Wright, Lee Trevino, and Tiger Woods (during the time he took lessons from Butch Harmon), helps you build a strong balanced foundation for swinging down at high speed, plus creates powerful leverage that, in turn, allows you to get the most out of your tee shots—and not simply in terms of power. This squat-action is a necessary conduit to delivering the club face squarely to the ball and hitting on-target shots. Furthermore, it is far easier to arrive in this position if you trigger the downswing with the right side. So, why aren't more instructors teaching right-handed golfers to depend more on their natural side, particularly during the most critical stage of the swing?

In answering this question, there is no doubt in my mind that I must come back to the lack of what I call "modernized instruction." Frankly, too many golf teachers are behind the times, out of touch with what's really going on. Many golf instructors simply accept that the so-called fundamentals governing the swing are evergreen in nature. Other instructors, except maybe just a few teachers ranked highly by *Golf* and *Golf Digest* magazines, are not curious enough to look outside the box and examine closely what the game's very best drivers have done or do to hit tee shots that fly far down the fairway. Other teaching professionals believe so wholeheartedly in their method (usually the very same one he or she employs when playing golf), that the natural course of action is to force it on the student. If the student doesn't "get it," the teacher simply tells the man, woman, junior, or senior player to practice more.

Alternatively, teachers tend to adopt a method that is the most popular at the moment. Right now, for example, golf instructors are teaching recreational players to "keep the arms and club in front of the body during the swing," just because these are the hot buzzwords used so often by top instructors and color commentators during televised golf events.

Golf teaching professionals will benefit from doing what

I've done in this book: analyze Michelle Wie's virtual flaw-less driver-swing technique and explain why a right-sided downswing works best.

It's very surprising to me that so few teachers have re-alized by now that a right-sided downswing action like Wie's is more natural and free, easier to repeat for the av-erage golfer, and requires less practice. It causes the arms and club to drop down into the ideal hitting slot, with the hands going along for the ride (instead of taking control and wrecking the swing), and the hinge in the right wrist is nicely maintained.

The hinged position of the right wrist might seem in-consequential to you; you might be under the impression that once the arms and club drop down, you should unhinge the wrist, then, a split second later, rotate the right forearm and right hand over the left forearm and left hand in the impact zone. If I'm right, this does not surprise me one bit. I say this because, in talking to amateur golfers around the country and around the globe, it is clear the typical recre-ational player has the wrong impression that early forearm rotation is a necessary fundamental for returning the club squarely to the ball at impact.

The average amateur also believes that the sooner you uncock the right wrist and release the club, the more snap and speed you'll create, and the harder you'll hit the ball. The truth is, the secret to power is delaying the release or "keeping the club away from the ball as long as possible,"

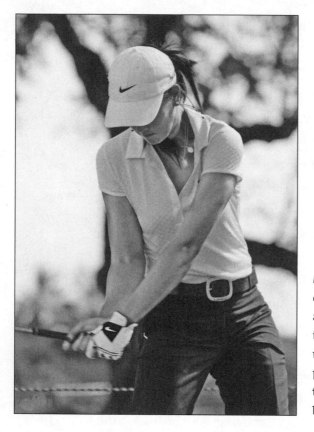

Michelle's right-sided downswing allows her arms and the club to drop into the ideal hitting slot, with the right wrist hinged, though poised to straighten and snap the club face squarely into the back of the ball at high speed.

which is what teacher Phil Ritson taught me and what I'm now convinced is one of Michelle Wie's power secrets.

Wie generates power by virtue of an active body and passive hands. Ritson calls this "rotation power." Specifically, Wie keeps her hands, arms, and right shoulder back during the downswing, rather than closer to the ball with what Ritson calls that "swing-wrecking over-the-top move" or "early hit."

It's a good idea, then, to look at both the black-and-white and color photographs of Michelle's downswing, and let the images of her delayed release and late hit form in your brain. That way, on the course, you will be much more likely to keep the club away from the ball until impact when the right wrist straightens and snaps the club face into the ball at maximum speed—in Wie's case, around 107 miles per hour, when hitting drives an average of 280 yards.

"By the time you have reached the impact zone, you will have rotated at least 80 percent of your weight onto the outside of your left foot," said Ritson in *Golf Your Way*, a book on which I collaborated with him in 1992.

"The remaining weight will be on the inside of your right foot, while the right heel is being pulled further off the ground by the force of the swing. Meanwhile, your head should remain steady behind the ball." (In Wie's case, her head is well back, about one foot behind the ball.)

Although I've cited numerous positions and the most vital links of the downswing, I want you to understand that, once triggered by the right side, the entire action is essentially reactive or reflexive. Said another way, once you spark the downward movement Wie-style, you will swing through the various positions with the ball merely getting in the way. The secret then is to hit up and through the ball instead of at it, by driving the lower body toward the target, keeping the head and upper body back away from the target, swinging at the highest possible speed while staying balanced, and letting Michelle Wie be your model.

As a prelude to discussing the post-impact positions, please heed my advice to practice the following simple Downswing-Trigger Drill, which will help you perfect your right-sided downswing triggers.

Step 1: Stand in front of a mirror in your driver address position.

Step 2: Swing the driver back to the top and stop.

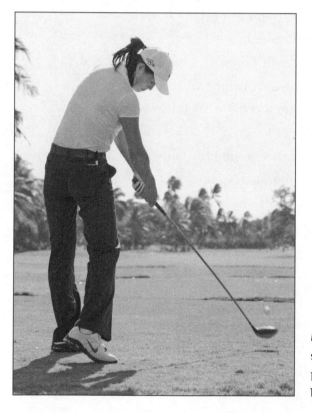

Michelle Wie arrives in the swing's moment-of-truth position: impact. Look and learn.

Step 3: Trigger the downswing by drawing the instep of your right foot downward and inward, pushing your right hip downward, and rotating your right knee inward, all in one piece simultaneously, so that your action is as rhythmic as Wie's.

Step 4: Hold the position for a few seconds, so that you can feel the sensation and look in the mirror to see what it looks like. The better you know your right-sided triggers, the more apt you will be to repeat them on the course and hit good drives—the Michelle Wie Way.

The Follow-Through and Finish Positions

Country club golfers I've spoken to about the swing wonder why it is so important to discuss post-impact positions—they argue that the ball has already been hit, so it makes no sense to be concerned about the look of the follow-through and finish positions.

I can well understand this viewpoint. Nevertheless, learning the physical elements of a technically correct Michelle-Wie-type follow-through and finish, and mentally "seeing" yourself arriving in these very same post-impact body positions, will help you employ a freewheeling downswing action that's vital to accelerating the club head through the ball at maximum speed. (*Note*: I mentioned post-impact "body" positions, and not club positions. I believe that if your body does an outstanding job of playing the lead role when swinging through impact, the club will successfully play an outstanding supporting role virtually automatically.)

Although I have been playing golf for 49 years, I remain curious about the golf swing. I'm always on the lookout for technical secrets that will ring a "that's it!" bell in my head, allow me to hit the ball more powerfully and accurately, and better relay the instructional message to players such as yourself through my books.

Recently, and strangely enough while researching a new art book I'm about to start writing, I discovered two paintings that to my absolute astonishment contained the best possible visual images for understanding the paramount positions of the golf swing's follow-through and finish positions.

When seeing the Henri Matisse painting, *Small Dancer Red Background* (circa 1937/1938), on page 281 of the book *Matisse* (edited by Jack Flam and published in 1990 by Park Lane), I truly could not believe my eyes, if you'll please excuse the cliché. That's because this work, though somewhat abstract, gives us more than a clue to what the body should do when swinging through impact. It clearly shows the most critical body positions of the early follow-through: lower body moving forward, upper body tilting back, arms extended. Offbeat I know, but I really urge you to look at this painting, because often a non-golf image will stick in

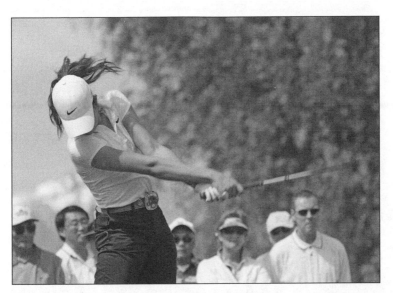

Michelle Wie in the early follow-through position (above), reminiscent of a painting by Henri Matisse, and in the late follow-through position (below).

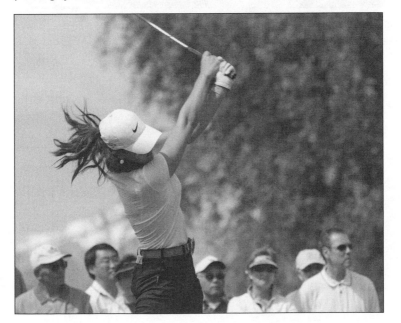

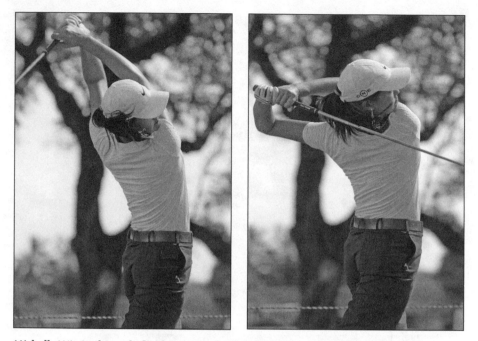

Michelle Wie in the early finish position (left), reminiscent of a painting by Agnolo Bronzino, and in the late finish position (right).

your mind much more strongly than a golf image, and thus leave a more lasting impression.

A month later into my research, I nearly fell off my chair when I came upon a beautiful piece by Agnolo Bronzino painted in 1545, during the Italian Mannerist Period. Called *An Allegory with Venus and Cupid*, this extraordinary and wonderful work shows a putto in the perfect early finish position, only instead of holding a golf club, the little boy is grasping a garland of roses. The boy's right shoulder has rotated under the chin, his left leg is stabilized, his right knee is rotated inward, all but the front toes of his right foot are off the ground, and his hands are high.

I found it quite ironic, indeed, that I should find these images, showing body positions that would make any top-ranked golf teacher proud, in an art book. All I could think of was this: Since Matisse is French and Bronzino Italian, maybe the visual messages contained in these paintings tell us that golf evolved from either the French game *Jeu de Mail* or the Italian game *Paganica*, as some golf historians believe, and was actually played in either of these countries earlier than on the links of Scotland.

As I leave you to ponder the evolution of the game Michelle Wie plays so well, let me just add this: It's true that golf, with its up and down cycles, imitates life, and that life imitates art.

MICHELLE WIE'S MASTERFUL DOWNSWING POSITIONS

Michelle triggers the downward swing movement by simultaneously putting pressure on her right foot, pushing the right hip downward, and turning the right knee inward.

Michelle's hips slide laterally early in the downswing, just as Hogan's did (though he has thrown a lot of golfers off, in the book *Five Lessons*, by focusing more on his downswing hip-clearing action). Sliding the hips, as opposed to turning them counterclockwise (clearing the hips) early in the downswing, will enhance the timing of your action.

Michelle's right shoulder moves down, her left shoulder up, paving the way for a strong upswing hit at impact.

Michelle's left leg braces late in the downswing, providing a firm axis to rotate her hips around and hit powerfully against.

Michelle's right wrist straightens due to centrifugal force working on the club head, and her right hand trigger finger helps her snap the club into the ball at high speed.

POWERFUL ADDED ATTRACTIONS

Use Michelle Wie's unique power-swing shotmaking techniques to become a more complete all-around golfer who hits a high percentage of quality shots

W hen playing golf at my own country club or visiting another course, I am amazed by the high number of golfers who lack the knowledge required for hitting a variety of shots. Particularly on weekends, when the course is the busiest, I witness golfers hit sky shots, fat shots, thin shots, shanks, topped drives, duck hooks and, of course, slice shots, then turn to their playing partner and ask, "What did I do wrong?"

The fact that the golf course looks like a circus sideshow saddens me, but frankly it also frustrates me. The main reason: I talk to average golfers all the time and although they complain about the state of their games, they rarely, if ever, sacrifice playing time for practice time.

To become good at golf, you must do a lot more than just hit a soft-draw drive far down the fairway—Michelle Wie's bread-and-butter shot. Educated golfers like Michelle and Tiger Woods prove that in order to shoot low scores you must evolve into a shotmaking virtuoso by disciplining yourself to take a series of lessons from your local golf professional or doing what some of the game's greatest shotmakers have done: Practice on your own with different clubs in your bag, constantly changing the position of the ball in your stance, opening then closing the club face, altering your weight distribution or the position of your hands, changing the speed of your swing, or shortening it.

To get you off to the right start and increase your repertoire of shots, I'm going to give you a crash course in shotmaking techniques by analyzing how Michelle Wie plays long and short shots—each require unique setup, backswing, and/or downswing principles and either sheer power or some form of body-club acceleration in order to hit.

Learn to hit the following shots and you'll not only impress other players in your regular weekend foursome, you'll proudly post a much lower score week after week.

Come with me to the lesson tee, so I can analyze how Michelle further applies power when hitting an array of shots during a round of golf, starting with the power-fade—a shot she sometimes hits off the tee on holes that curve right, or "dogleg," to wind the ball around the corner and leave herself an easier, shorter shot into the green.

Power-Fade Driver Technique

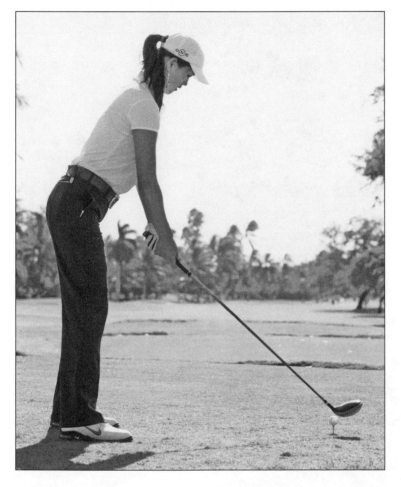

Jockeying your body into an open position is critical when setting up to play a power-fade drive off the tee.

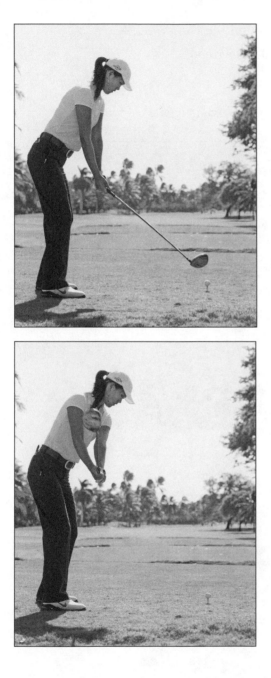

When taking the club away, like Michelle Wie is doing in the two photographs at left, and swinging to the top in the three sequence photographs at right, you will feel as if you are wrongly directing the club outside the target line. That's okay. Due to the open setup, you are merely swinging the club parallel to your feet and body lines, running left of the target, precisely along the line on which the ball will begin flying, before curving or fading right.

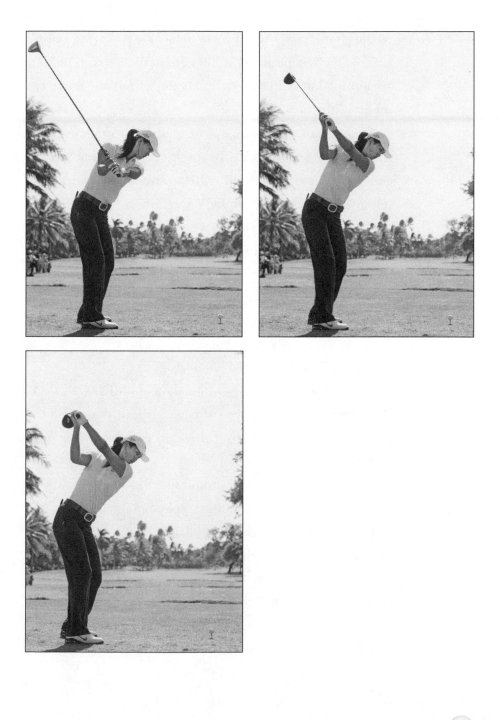

In the photograph showing Michelle Wie jockeying herself into the address position, you'll note her feet and shoulders are aiming left of the target, at an area of fairway down the center of the fairway.

To program this unique power-fade shot into your own address, follow Michelle's example of setting up "open," and stand closer to the ball with a more erect posture. The more you want the ball to fade, the farther left you should aim your feet and body. However, always aim the club face directly at that area of fairway where you ultimately want the ball to land.

Due to the open setup, you will feel in the takeaway like you are swinging the club outside the target line when, in fact, you are simply swinging along a path that's square to your body line, just like Michelle does.

If you look at the photographs showing Michelle's backswing, you'll see she appears to be "laying the club off," when in fact she's swinging the club parallel to her open stance.

On the downswing, you should feel like you're swinging across the target line. Even in the photograph showing Michelle in the through-impact position, it appears she's done that. The fact is she swings the club down along a line parallel to her "open" feet and body. Why? You want the ball to start flying down the center of the fairway, then curve to the right around the dogleg. You'll accomplish this goal if you set up open, position the club face square to your final landing spot, and swing back and through along imaginary lines running across your feet and body.

The shot you hit will fly fast off the club face, rise quickly, then level off into a penetrating trajectory as it fades back to its final target (an area of fairway down the right side), allowing you to "cut the dogleg," as good golfers say.

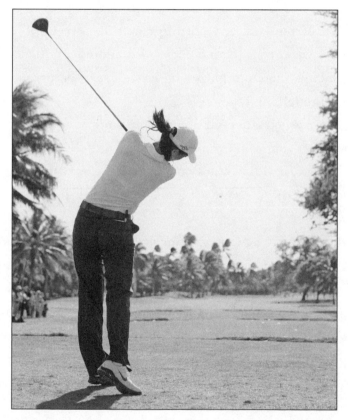

Swinging the club down and through your open body lines will help promote the desired fade-spin you want to be imparted on the ball at impact.

Fairway-Metal Power-Play Shot

Whenever the ball is sitting down slightly and you are quite a long way from the green, a lofted fairway-metal club is an excellent choice of "stick" to use to hit a powerful recovery shot, provided you follow Wie's example.

The two most important elements of the setup are playing the ball back in the stance, setting the hands slightly ahead of the ball, and putting about 55 percent of your body's weight on the left foot. This address position will promote a more upright swing as well as a sharper down-and-through hit.

You are going to need to put some more oomph into this shot than you would when playing a normal fairway shot. Therefore, it's important that you turn the body fully while keeping the swing compact for added control and enhanced balance.

On the way down, use your right hip, right knee, and right foot triggers to encourage the club to drop down into the ideal hitting slot. Once it does, start clearing your left hip to open up a clear path for the club to swing along. As soon as you feel your left leg start to brace, turn your right hip counterclockwise. This right-side thrust action will add power to your shot and boost you through into the finish.

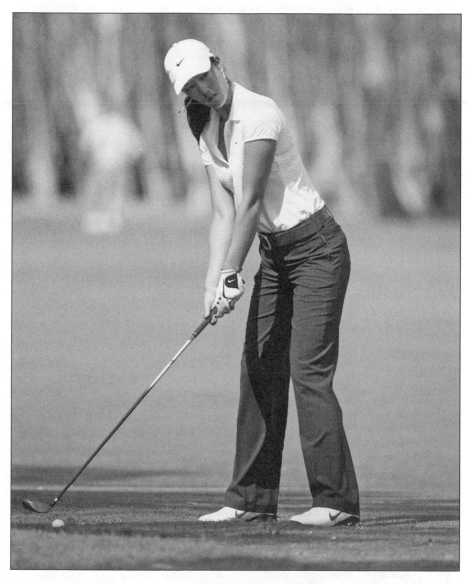

When the ball is down, you need to play the ball back in the stance, as Michelle does here, to promote a slightly more upright swing than normal and a sharper hit at impact.

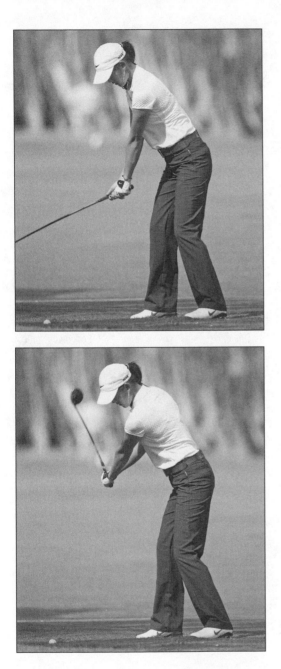

The two photographs at left and the two photographs at right show how important it is to swing the club back and up on a steep plane to the three-quarter point. Like Michelle Wie, you are then poised to hit down and through the ball powerfully and hit a good shot from this type of lie.

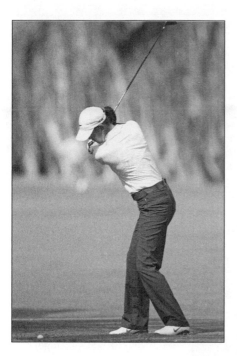

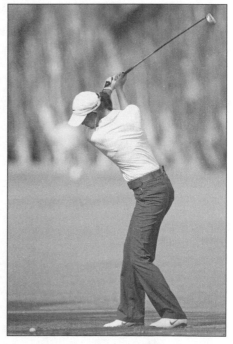

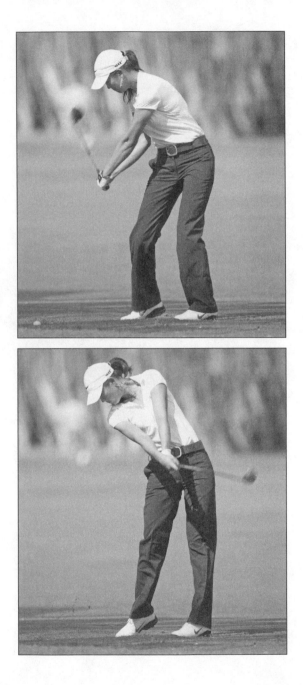

In playing a fairway-metal shot from this type lie, Michelle Wie swings the club sharply down into the impact zone (but not on an overly steep angle), and maintains good arm extension to ensure a low, powerful flight trajectory of the golf ball.

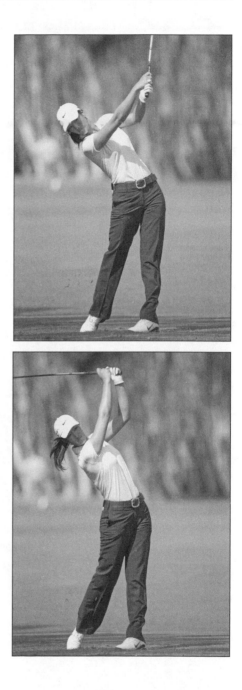

Michelle swings through fluidly into the finish, proving that her right-side triggers are on full thrust; this is necessary in the hitting area in order to pinch the ball out of the grass and propel it far down the fairway or all the way to the green.

Long-Iron Power-Play

Golfers are afraid of long irons, even when facing a shot off a clean fairway lie. That's because these clubs feature such a small degree of loft compared to the short irons that the average player thinks he or she has little chance of solidly hitting the ball into the air.

The address and backswing keys for playing this shot are similar to those required for hitting a driver the way Michelle Wie does. In short, you should set the feet wide apart at address to establish a strong base that will allow you to swing the club along a wide arc and support your powerful motion.

The downswing is another matter, requiring a different swing than what's used by Michelle Wie when she hits a driver. Rather than making contact on the upswing, you want to create a long flat spot on your downswing by swinging through the ball with the club moving low to the ground in a streamlined fashion. Furthermore, in order to promote clean contact and send the ball flying high into the air so that it lands softly on the green, you must follow Michelle's example of freely clearing the hips, extending the arms through the hit zone, and accelerating into a full finish position.

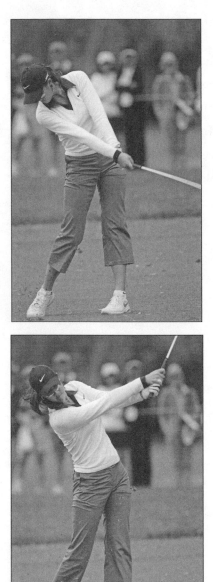

The secret to hitting powerful long-iron shots is making a streamlined follow-through action (left) then swinging upward into a high finish with the lower body driving forward, the upper body rocking back (right).

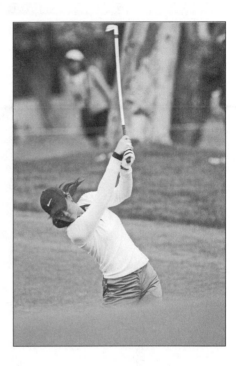

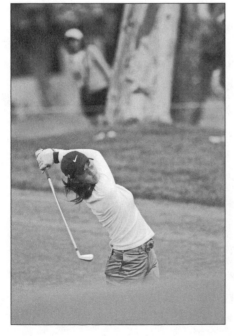

Power-Iron Tee Shot

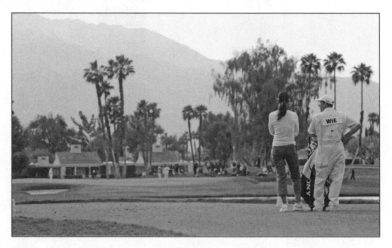

On a par-3 hole, where you have the best chance of scoring birdie, the tendency is to rush. Instead, follow Michelle's example of being deliberate yet decisive during your pre-shot routine. Think before you act, but don't spend too much time thinking.

On this par-3 hole, Michelle Wie proves that she is a very patient player, taking time to talk to her caddie about the distance to the hole, the speed and firmness of the green, and any wind that might influence her choice of club. You, too, need to resolve any playing condition issues, on your own or with a playing partner or caddie. In order to make a strong, free swing and hit an on-target middle- or short-iron shot, there can be absolutely no doubt whatsoever in your mind about the club you intend to play the shot with.

To hit an on-line power-iron shot that flies toward the hole and lands very softly on the green, you need to set your feet, knees, hips, and shoulders square to the target line.

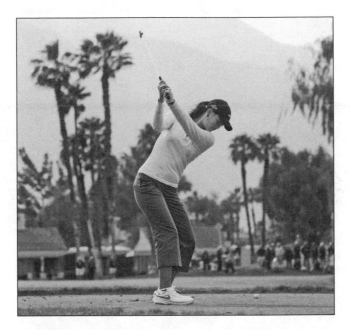

When playing a power-iron tee shot, your backswing should be
compact and controlled, just like Michelle Wie's.

The face of the club should also be square—and pointing
directly at your target.

Swing back until you feel that your weight is balanced on
your right foot and leg and also keep the backswing compact
for added control. An overly long backswing can negatively
affect the rhythm of your swing, thereby preventing you
from staying balanced and synchronizing the movement of
the body with the movement of the club.

Let your right side spark your downswing action, then
once you feel the weight shift to your left foot and leg, accelerate your arms through the impact zone.

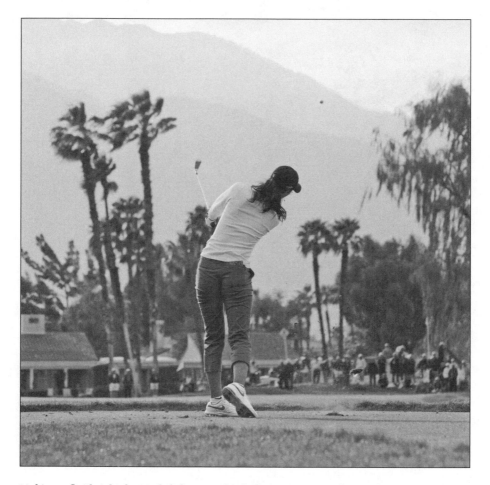

Making a fluid right foot to left foot weight shift action is critical to swinging the club down correctly and hitting a solid on-line power-iron tee shot, as Michelle proves in these two photographs.

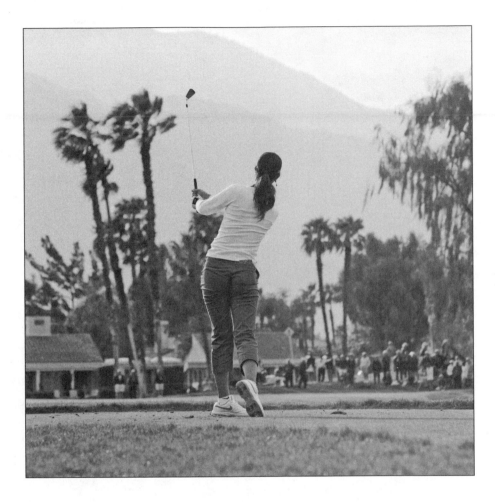

Power-Iron Shot Off Uphill Lie

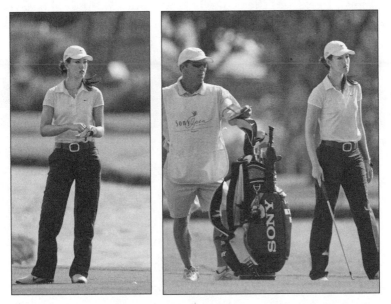

Before setting up to play a power-iron shot off an uphill lie, look toward the green and determine where it's best to land the ball (left) then select a stronger club (i.e., a six-iron instead of a seven-iron) for the distance at hand (right).

When you face an uphill lie, take the time to assess the distance to the hole and surrounding hazards, as Michelle Wie does. You always want to maintain a positive attitude, and at the same time determine whether it's best to land the ball on the green well beyond the flag or in front of the green, a short distance from the hole. When choosing a club, you also have to take into consideration that off an uphill lie the effective loft of the club is increased; compensate by choosing a stronger club than you would normally when playing a level shot from the same distance. For example, choose a six-iron instead of a seven-iron.

Loss of balance is something else you must guard against, so when addressing the ball increase the flex in your knees and tilt your body to your right, so that you stand as perpendicular to the slope as you comfortably can and, essentially, give yourself a level lie.

Make a super-controlled compact backswing, as Michelle does, making sure to keep your right knee braced and your head practically dead still.

The major keys to attaining clean club-face-to-ball contact are driving the arms and club downward then swinging the club along the contour of the slope with steady acceleration through the impact area.

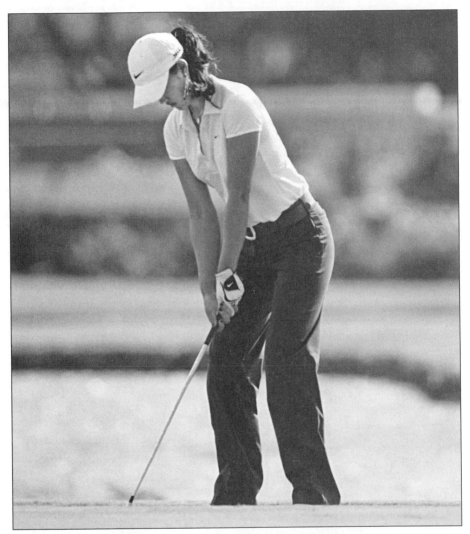

Bending more at the knees and tilting your body slightly to your right—two important
address keys when playing an uphill power-iron shot.

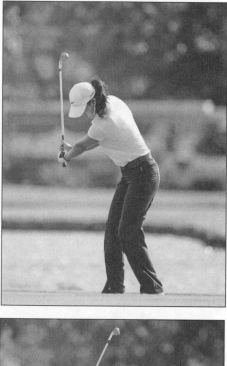

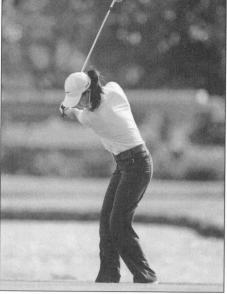

Following Michelle's example of keeping the right knee braced and the backswing shorter (left) will allow you to be readied to make your power-play off an uphill lie.

In order to make clean and powerful contact with the ball off an uphill lie, let the club follow the contour of the slope as Michelle Wie illustrates in the photographs at right.

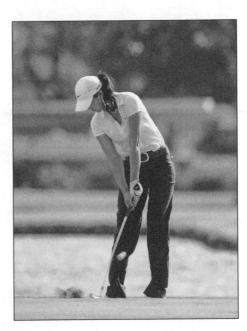

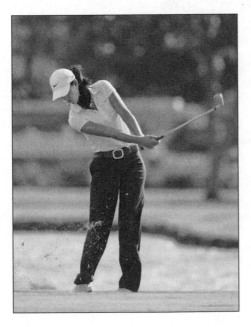

Power-Iron Shot Off Side-Hill Lie

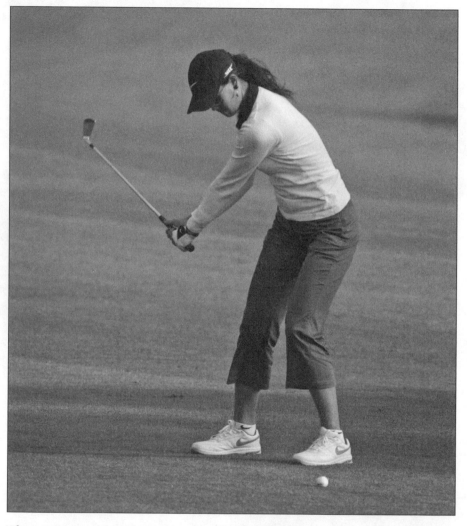

When preparing to hit a power-iron shot off a side-hill lie and the ball is above your feet, it's important to first rehearse the early set wrist action needed when playing this shot, as Michelle Wie illustrates above.

Anytime the ball is above your feet, the tendency is to swing on too flat a path and plane. This fault causes the club to become trapped behind your body on the downswing and ultimately triggers a weak shot hit right of target. So, before setting up, it's a good idea to practice an early set of the right wrist. This pre-swing rehearsal helps you get the feel for the right type action and guard against making an overly rounded swing.

On the backswing, swing the club back to the three-quarter position, with your arms playing the lead role.

When swinging down, generate power in the impact zone by unhinging your right wrist, so that you accelerate your arms and the club through the ball.

Tailoring the Tip

This type of side-hill lie will make the ball turn a little from right to left and fly faster off the club face. Therefore, choose either one of the following strategies to compensate for the degree of slope and curve of the ball:

1. Choose one club less than normal for the distance at hand (i.e., a seven-iron instead of a six-iron) to compensate for the "hot" ball flight, and aim the club and your body right of target to allow for the ball's turning-left pattern. Next, simply swing.

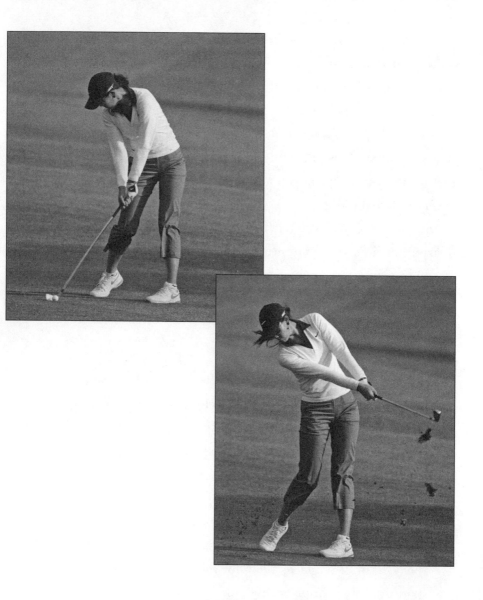

These three photographs show the vital importance of letting the arms accelerate the club into impact then through the ball, when playing a power-iron shot off a side-hill lie with the ball above your feet.

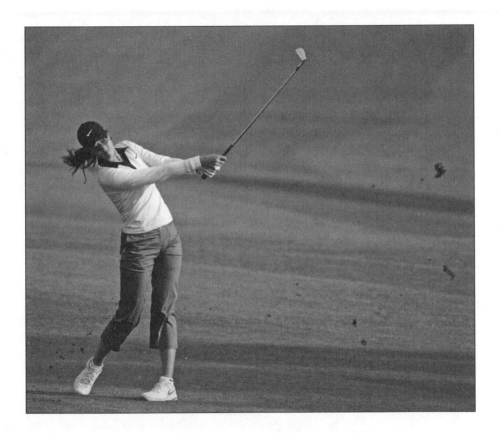

2. Set your body square to the target with the club face open (the more severe the side-hill slope, the more you should open the club's face), and make your normal swing.

Power-Lift Iron Shot

Whenever you face a shot off a lie in an area of thin grass, on or off the fairway, and you need to hit the ball extra-high to carry a tree in front of you or land the ball extra-softly on a firm green, follow these instructions, based on what I learned watching Michelle Wie in action:

In setting up, put about 55 percent of your weight on your right foot and position your hands behind the ball slightly.

Swing the club back on an upright plane, stopping at the three-quarter point.

In swinging down, rotate your lower body toward the target while keeping your head and upper body weight behind the ball and accelerating your arms.

Tailoring the Tip

The shotmaking technique described above can cause you to increase the effective loft of the club at impact. Therefore, if the shot is, say, 150 yards, seven-iron distance for most golfers, select a six-iron instead. But, by all means, practice so that you can make the right club-choice adjustments suited to your own game.

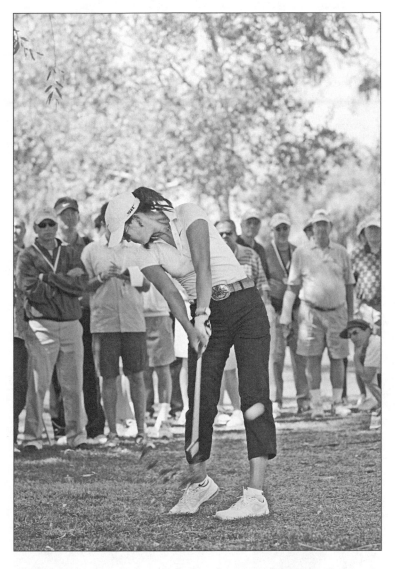

In order to pick the ball cleanly off a patch of threadbare grass then propel it into the air like Michelle does here, tilt your head and upper body back through impact, while accelerating your arms and the club through the ball.

Power-Punch

It's true that the worst strategy you should depend on when playing a shot into a wind is to swing fast. The reason: You will lose your balance and control of the shot. The irony: Golfers who know this tend to swing so slowly that they fail to propel the ball all the way to the hole.

Michelle Wie is the ideal model for learning how to handle a headwind. From what I've observed, her tempo is upbeat, but her rhythm is smooth and controlled. More important, rather than swing the club down on a steep angle, the path of her downswing is quite shallow.

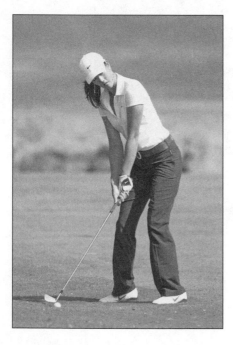

Three important technical "musts" for hitting a power-punch shot: playing the ball back in a slightly closed stance (left), swinging into the ball from an inside path (right top), and striving to match the low finish of Michelle Wie (right bottom).

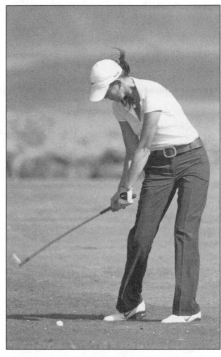

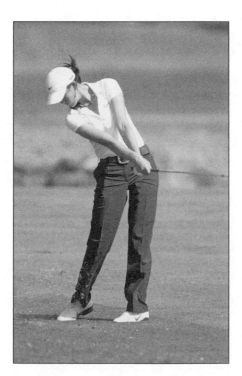

In order to hit a low, controlled shot that "cheats" the wind, set up with the ball back slightly in your stance and your feet in a "closed" position (right foot back a little farther from the target line than the left foot), swing the club back inside the target line, swing the club through on a shallow path, and finish low.

Power-Spin Shot

Many recreational golfers that I speak to believe imparting backspin on the ball is something that only a top profes-

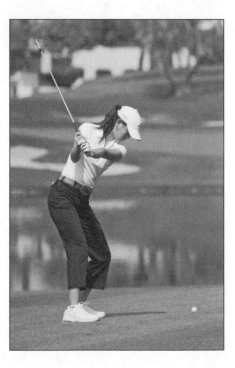

Critical keys to hitting a power-spin short- or middle-iron shot: swinging the club along the correct plane (left), using your right-side triggers to help you drive the club powerfully into the ball (right top), and accelerating the club into the follow-through (right bottom).

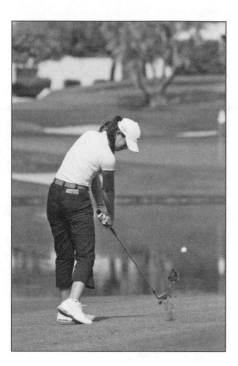

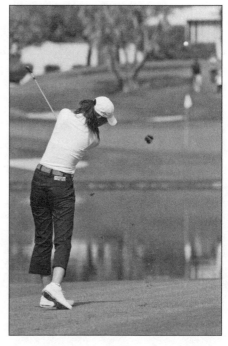

sional can accomplish. Strangely enough, getting the ball to land beyond the flagstick and spin back a few yards toward the cup does not require a Herculean effort on the part of the player. In fact, provided you heed the following technical recipe, based on what Michelle Wie does in action, it's really quite easy to hit a spinning wedge shot.

At address, play the ball back in your stance with 60 percent of your weight on your left foot and your hands a couple of inches ahead of the ball. Also, when gripping the club, be sure that the back of your left hand is square to the club face.

Swing the club back along the plane established by the angle of the club shaft at address, allowing your right wrist to hinge quite early in the takeaway.

Swing the club down into the ball, keeping the club on plane and the back of the left hand square at impact. Accelerate your hands, arms, and the club into the follow-through.

If you did everything right, in particular contacting the ball before hitting the turf, you'll take a divot and see the ball sailing high in the air on its way to the target beyond the flag, before spinning back "stiff" to the hole.

Author JOHN ANDRISANI was a longtime senior instruction editor of *Golf Magazine*. Best known for writing *The Tiger Woods Way* and collaborating with golf instructor Jim Hardy on *The Plane Truth for Golfers*, Andrisani plays off a six handicap at Pasadena Yacht & Country Club in Gulfport, Florida.

Photographer YASUHIRO TANABE's photography has been showcased in numerous golf books and golf magazines.